Praise for *No Ap*

A *New York Times Book Review* Editors' Choice Staff Pick
One of the *Texas Observer*'s "10 Texas Books
We Loved in 2017"

"Engrossing. . . . Pearson's vivid writing sometimes lulls you into the trance of a good story—character, voice, plot, conflict—but there's always the sucker punch at the end to remind you of the gruesome endpoint of the American healthcare system. . . . Her literary skill is apparent in her book. Her courage, honesty and doggedness are evident on every page."   —Danielle Ofri, *New York Times Book Review*

"*No Apparent Distress* is filled with the moving stories of a medical student's journey providing health care at the margins of American life. Rachel Pearson shines a spotlight on the brutal inequalities present within our healthcare system."
—Damon Tweedy, MD, author of *Black Man in a White Coat*

"Rachel Pearson comes from a hard place. In her memoir *No Apparent Distress* she tells the story of a Texas hospital that has been flattened by a hurricane and is being rebuilt—literally rebuilt—around her and her colleagues while they pursue their medical training. Working at a clinic for the poor and uninsured teaches Pearson the empathy she will need to cultivate if she expects to act as an effective advocate for her patients. It also teaches her about the inequities and injustices of the American health care system, and the labor of love required of anyone who decides to pursue the practice of medicine in this country."
—Judy Melinek, MD, and T. J. Mitchell, coauthors of the *New York Times* best-selling memoir *Working Stiff: Two Years, 262 Bodies, and the Making of a Medical Examiner*

"A notable contribution to the medical *bildungsroman*."
—*The BMJ* Medical Humanities blog

NO APPARENT DISTRESS

*A Doctor's Coming-of-Age on the
Front Lines of American Medicine*

Rachel Pearson, MD

W. W. NORTON & COMPANY
Independent Publishers Since 1923
New York   London

No patient's real name is used in this book without such patient's express consent. Even then, certain potentially identifying details have been changed. The names, physical features, and other potentially identifying characteristics of many other people in this book also have been changed.

The views and opinions expressed in this book are solely those of the author. They are not and do not reflect the views or opinions of any organization or institution with which she is affiliated or has been affiliated or of anyone else employed by or affiliated with such organization or institution.

For information about permission to reproduce selections from this book, write to Permissions, W. W. Norton & Company, Inc., 500 Fifth Avenue, New York, NY 10110

For information about special discounts for bulk purchases, please contact W. W. Norton Special Sales at specialsales@wwnorton.com or 800-233-4830

Manufacturing by LSC Communications, Harrisonburg
Book design by Lovedog Studio
Production manager: Louise Mattarelliano

Library of Congress Cataloging-in-Publication Data

Names: Pearson, Rachel, 1983– author.
Title: No apparent distress : a doctor's coming-of-age on the front lines of American
   medicine / Rachel Pearson.
Description: First edition. | New York : W.W. Norton & Company, [2017] |
   Includes index.
Identifiers: LCCN 2016055803 | ISBN 9780393249248 (hardcover)
Subjects: | MESH: Students, Medical | Education, Medical | Healthcare
   Disparities | Health Care Rationing | Socioeconomic Factors | United States |
   Personal Narratives
Classification: LCC RA418 | NLM W 18 | DDC 362.1—dc23
LC record available at https://lccn.loc.gov/2016055803

ISBN 978-0-393-35585-7 pbk.

W. W. Norton & Company, Inc.
500 Fifth Avenue, New York, N.Y. 10110
www.wwnorton.com

W. W. Norton & Company Ltd.
15 Carlisle Street, London W1D 3BS

1 2 3 4 5 6 7 8 9 0

For my father

NOTE

This is a work of nonfiction that includes some stories about people who have been my patients and the patients of my friends. Whether or not I was able to ask a particular patient for permission to use his or her story, I have changed details that might make that person identifiable. I have done the same with some of the health care professionals and medical students whose stories I tell.

We live in a time of hardening of hearts. Please don't ask me why. I don't know why God hardened the heart of the pharaoh. All I know is that right now, we are living in that time.

—Michael Thomas Jackson,
lay minister of St. Vincent's House, 2015

Any man's death diminishes me, because I am involved in mankind.

—John Donne,
Devotions upon Emergent Occasions, *1624*

NO APPARENT DISTRESS

PROLOGUE

MR. ROSE HAS THIS PAIN. HE HAS THIS PAIN IN HIS STOM-
ach . . . *man, right here in my stomach!* . . . and it comes and it goes but
it's been there for four weeks, he guesses, though he's not really sure
because he was living with his sister and then her husband started
using and wanted to put some of his own sorry-ass friends on the
couch, excuse the French, Doc, but the things she goes through, it's
plain wrong—the pain? No, he doesn't take anything for it. He tried
everything. His sister gave him some Norco. He's got this pain, and
yeah, there's a bad odor in his mouth. Well, he eats whatever, if he's at
his sister's house he eats maybe a TV dinner, or if he's with his cousin,
sometimes they'll barbecue. He doesn't get to pick and choose, you
see. Sometimes he doesn't eat for a while. And the food is getting
stuck in his throat, like right here. No, there's nowhere he lives on
a regular basis. He doesn't have a telephone number. But he's been
eating less and less because . . . this pain.

I liked Mr. Rose right off, maybe in part because I met him before
I learned the term "poor historian." Later, when he showed up at the
ER sweating and moaning, with his heart rhythm gone bad and his
blood so thin it barely carried enough oxygen to keep him walking,
the medical student who saw him there would say to me, "I wish
you'd've been there when he came in, because you know his whole

history. You're like his primary care doctor. And it's hard to get a story out of Mr. Rose . . . he's such a poor historian."

And when we finally knew about the cancer that had been fermenting in his belly all those weeks, when we saw the CT scan that showed a mass the size of two grapefruits in his belly and I realized it had been there *and I never felt it* . . . I would rack back through his story searching for the thing that would've told me how fast he was dying. And it was there: my mistake. The mistake for which I will never be forgiven, because the person who could've forgiven me was gone before I knew how to ask.

But I get ahead of myself. I, too, can be a poor historian.

CHAPTER 1

IN 1981, TWO DAYS AFTER MY OLDER BROTHER MATTHEW was born, my father sawed off the tip of his index finger. He was building an extension on to the Airstream trailer that my family was living in, in a clearing on a tract of land in the East Texas woods. Dad was working in a hurry, because my grandmother was on the way down from Arkansas to meet her first grandchild, and Dad wanted her to be comfortable. He must have been tired, too. He was running a two-by-eight into the table saw when the blade caught his fingertip and shredded it.

So Dad came hollering out of the sheet-metal workshop that still stands on that land. Blood streamed off his elbow. My mother had never seen him panic before, and she hasn't since. She ran across the cleared field to hail my great-uncle Arnold, who wrapped Dad's hand in a T-shirt and drove him down the dirt road that branches onto another dirt road that leads to Farm-to-Market Road 1097, and on to the hospital in Conroe. It was May, and wildflowers were still blooming along the way—eternal thanks to Lady Bird Johnson.

The doctors at the hospital patched Dad up, and he did not let the wound slow him down much. He finished the extension before my grandmother arrived. The finger healed.

By the time I was born two years later, it was clear that my brother was a bright child. My father would point down at us with his middle finger, keeping the sawed-short index finger bent in the way he still does, and say, "Reta, how are we ever going to send these kids to college?"

It was a question that had no answer—not in 1983. But it was important to my father, who did not graduate from college. He and my mother made a deal that he would support her through college if she stayed home for a few years while Matt and I were small. So I have early memories of coloring in the back of college classrooms and accompanying my mom's ornithology class on a field trip. She eventually became a high school biology teacher, and Dad never wavered in his expectation that Matt and I would have college degrees.

All I can remember of that trailer is sunlight filtered through the tall pines and beaming in a back window, where it caught dust motes. The floor slanted a little bit.

Shortly after I was born, Dad built a sawmill. He cleared land, and sawed the pine trees into boards. He built us a house on the land he'd cleared, and Mom used her student loans to get a dishwasher. I grew up loving the sweet smell of pine sawdust and the enticing soft piles of it that built up near the sawmill—good to smell, but too itchy to jump in. Dad built us furniture. He built me a step stool, stilts, and a play kitchen with working cabinets. He built the table I am writing at now. He built the bunk bed that my brother and I shared in a room with rainbow curtains that my mother sewed. We would leap off the top bunk into refrigerator boxes that my dad brought home for us from his construction jobs.

THE SUMMER I TURNED ELEVEN, my family moved to Port Aransas, Texas, home to three thousand hardy souls. Port Aransas is on Mustang Island, a small barrier island about midway down the Texas coast between the Louisiana and Mexico borders. To be specific, we moved to the Mustang Island RV Resort, and took up a spot in our camper while my dad and my brother, who was thirteen then, built us a house on a property down the road.

The camper was cozy. It didn't extend much beyond the bed of my dad's pickup truck. There was a loft space that went above the cab of the pickup, and my brother and I slept there. Below, there was a tiny kitchen and a table that folded down into a bed, where my parents slept at night. There was also a miniature toilet, but we mostly just used the restroom at the RV park. We cooked outside on the grill a lot, and ate on the picnic table at our spot. My mom says this was one of the happiest years she can remember. So if you can imagine living in a tiny camper in an RV park in Texas with a thirteen-year-old and an eleven-year-old and two small dogs, I guess this tells you something about my family. We get along.

Some of the happiness was lost on me, though, because by the time we moved to Port Aransas I had grown into an awkward child. Everyone will tell you that they were awkward in junior high, but I was a special case. For one thing, God had graced me with a set of those teeth that drugstores sell around Halloween, labeled "farmer teeth" or "hick teeth." One of my top teeth stuck out of the gum at a ninety-degree angle to the rest of my teeth. Two were twisted all the way around. My family got insured to the hilt by the time we moved to Port Aransas—Mom was teaching by then, and my dad got a job as an electrician at the University of Texas Marine Science Institute, which happens to be on Mustang Island. Consequently, I got braces.

The braces were the first hit on my junior high awkwardness regime. My wicked orthodontist prescribed a thing called a Haas device, that literally broke my upper palate so that all my teeth could fit in my head. Then he had me wrap two rubber bands around each brace. The rubber bands would pop off randomly and fly across the room. But luckily they started controlling my teeth.

I was largely left to my own devices when it came to fashion and grooming, with the sole exception being that I was not allowed to shave my legs. I don't know where I would've done it, anyway, because there was no bathtub in the trailer park. I would roll out of my sleeping bag sometime after my mom had left to commute to work, perform my perfunctory ablutions in the trailer park bathroom, and bicycle off to school on my prized possession: an awesome purple Diamondback bike. The clothes that I chose for myself—purple high-tops, a T-shirt I loved with sparkly papayas all over it, a purple windsuit—made me look like a cross between a Florida retiree and a bowl of fruit. And then there were the glasses. We were not the kind of family that could buy new glasses every time their two myopic preteens broke theirs. Instead, my father used his natural ingenuity and his skills as an electrician to solder my glasses back together. Over the course of the year, the lump of solder at the bridge of my nose got bigger and bigger.

When I got ready for school, I would brush my hair. But I would brush only the parts I could see, next to my face. It didn't occur to me to brush the back. And so gradually, over time, a huge rat's nest built up in the back of my head. It would be an insult to dreadlocks to call this a dreadlock. It was just a plum-sized knot of tangled, splitting hair. I hid it pretty effectively in my ponytail. Dad had always done my hair when I was younger, but in Port Aransas he was at work by the time I woke up. My mother might've noticed it anyway and combed it out if she hadn't been leaving at seven a.m. to commute to work, getting home around six p.m., and then cooking dinner before doing lesson plans and falling asleep. My parents' lack of attention to my appearance fell somewhere between feminist resistance to social norms about girls' appearance and benign neglect. So I grew up without any complexes about my body, but I certainly had a rat's nest. Sometimes I would reach my hand back and touch it, and it seemed so large and intractable and awful that I would just pull my hand back and pretend that it didn't exist.

Imagine me then: the double-banded braces, the soldered-together glasses, the hairy legs and knotted hair and trailer park grooming. I was not cool. Miraculously, though, I loved myself. In pictures from back then, I am grinning through my metal mouth, with my arms around the other awkward girls who took me into their fold.

One of those girls was Jennifer, whose family had a condo and a swimming pool on the island. Frankly, Jennifer's parents forced her to hang out with me. They thought I had moxie, and that I would be a good influence on shy Jennifer. So Jennifer and I formed a solidarity based on board games and the music of Queen, and over Christmas break her parents invited me to go on their annual skiing trip.

The skiing trip was my first real introduction to how the other half lives. I wrote postcards home detailing all of this: *They gave us peanuts on the airplane, but they were not honey roasted. They were salted. In the ski lodge, I paid two dollars for hot cocoa and they gave me extra marshmallows. My glasses broke so I'm wearing my sports glasses. I fell a fair distance down the mountain and broke both my legs. Just kidding!* And one night, beside the crackling ski lodge fire, Jennifer's mother sat down and combed the rat's nest out of my hair.

IT TOOK A YEAR OR SO for my family to build the house. We built it on afternoons and weekends, because Dad was working at the Marine Science Institute down the street. He kept that job for fifteen years, because it enabled us to have great insurance and he could benefit from the teacher retirement system. But he still says that it was a waste of his life in so many ways—digging ditches at age fifty, replacing light switches. He was a man who could design a house and build it from the ground up, who built a giant robot in his free time and then used it to make me a life-sized wooden velociraptor skeleton for my birthday. His creativity and his skills weren't much called for at his money job. "I never want you to have to work like that, not for insurance," he's told me.

I'm safe in my profession, but Dad still wants my brother to go back to school, to have all the chances that Dad never did. Sometimes I argue the point with him—college no longer guarantees a good job. But mostly I let it drop. I study; I am grateful.

The house is on stilts—big salt-resistant creosote-soaked pilings that seep sticky black in the heat—so floodwaters from a hurricane could pass underneath. (God forbid.) On every level, the floor and roof are secured with dozens and dozens of hurricane ties: *L*-shaped bits of metal that take eight nails each. Hammering hurricane ties was my job, and I hated it. Matt turned from a pudgy kid into a strong and lanky teenager the year we were building, hanging from the house frame forty feet up as he helped with everything: the framing, the wiring, the cabinets, the painting, the roof. Our neighbor did the shingles. Mom hammered, kept the workers fed and supplied with sweet iced tea, and supported the family with her teaching job. I helped lay the flooring when we graduated from painted plywood floors to varnished pine. Matt still works construction in the off-season from commercial fishing; last year he texted me a picture of him siding a house in six-foot-deep snow in Alaska.

DAD'S QUESTION about how they would send us to college was answered by the government: Matt and I both got full scholarships to the University of Texas at Austin, under a program that no longer exists. It was the best school I could imagine, and the only school I applied to. It was perfect.

The first two summers of college, I went home and worked for Dad. Dad had a big project, renovating twenty-six tiny abandoned cottages in the middle of Port Aransas. So my brother and I drove home from Austin in the beat-up Ford F-250 we shared, and spent the summers ripping out old plumbing, patching plaster, and hanging drywall. We worked in the heat of a South Texas summer, and everything we did had to be repeated twenty-six times. I liked the work. Matt had done plenty of construction work before, but I had never had work that felt so solid: I would work all day, and see in the evening what I had done. I began to understand why my father loved carpentry, and to get a glimpse of how creative that work could be, if you had the skills.

I was unskilled, however, so most of what I did was grunt labor. I spent some afternoons sweating under heavy plastic rain gear while

I power washed old paint off the concrete walls; tiny bits of concrete would blast back at me hard enough to have left bruises if it weren't for the rain gear. I decided to call Dad on the cell phone. He was supervising from afar while he worked his electrician job.

"It's like two hundred degrees under this rain gear," I told Dad. "I could faint."

"Bah," he said. "Drink some Gatorade." Like his own father before him, Dad has always believed that children are best utilized for manual labor, and that a significant benefit of hiring one's children is that you don't have to offer worker's compensation or supply safety devices. He did keep the cooler full of Gatorade, though.

The cottages had been on the transient highway for years, and not everyone was happy that we were developing them. One man left behind a mountain of trash when he evacuated a cottage he'd been squatting in. Another expressed his displeasure by killing a possum and smearing its guts all over the freshly hung drywall. We hung it again.

Matt and I spent one week ripping out the old toilets and carrying them across the property for storage. Dad insisted that these were "valuable antique toilets," built before water-conservation laws limited the number of gallons that could flow from a tank. He was going to sell these valuable toilets on eBay.

That week, I found that the bonds of civilization are strong but odd: Even though there had been no water running in the cottages for years, people had continued to shit in the dry toilets. Matt and I would flush them with bleach and water from the hose, then wrench off the bolts connecting the toilets to the floor. When we heaved them up, though, bleach water with traces of feces would splash out on my socks from the goose neck inside the toilets.

I called my dad on the cell phone. "Dad," I said. "I think we should abandon the toilets."

"Those are valuable antique toilets, Rach," he said.

"There's shit on my socks, Dad. Transient people's shit is splashing all over my socks."

"Use more bleach," he said.

I would like to state for the record that the valuable antique toilets were never sold on eBay. They stayed in an unused unit until Dad realized that it would be too much trouble to sell them, and then they went into a Dumpster.

That summer, my father started a tradition of cornering me in the evenings to have long conversations about my future. It was a sort of collaborative pipe dreaming, with both of us reveling in the opportunities that were open for me. In those conversations I could feel how wrapped I was in his love, and also the weight of my own life and how much it meant to him. Usually, Dad would encourage me to take premed classes, and I would refuse. "You could just get the basics now, kiddo, in case one day you want to apply," he'd say. "You never know. You'd be a great doctor." But back then I wanted to be a writer.

One evening, our conversation turned to marriage. I was sitting on the countertop in our kitchen, and the lights were dim. Dad's theories about my marriageability included suggesting that I shave my legs and stop being so particular. (I was twenty.) "What are you looking for?" he asked.

"Well, I guess I'd like to marry somebody like me," I said. "With a good education."

Dad quietly looked down. "Rachel, you never know," he said. "One of those guys without a college degree might surprise you."

I flushed, and stared down at the kitchen floor, which I had helped Dad install—covering the old painted plywood floor with real oak—in junior high. The oak was still golden, though scuffed from years of boots and heels, scratched by the toenails of two generations of dogs.

"I didn't mean . . . ," I began. I couldn't finish.

"It's okay," Dad said.

CHAPTER 2

IT WAS ABORTION THAT CONVINCED ME THAT MY DAD WAS right, and I should go into medicine. Not any abortion I had, but working in an abortion clinic. This is not a story I tell often.

The February after my last year of college, I got a job as a patient advocate at a clinic. When I arrived there for the first time, I thought, *It will look like I'm getting an abortion.* Then I shrugged and went in. I was twenty-two and had just gotten the news that I'd been accepted into the master of fine arts program in creative writing at Columbia. I needed money for the move to New York City, so I'd applied for a job as a patient advocate.

At my interview, the clinic leader pointed out that the clinic strives to be respectful of every patient.

"Of course," I said.

"I mean," she said, "we really try to be kind."

"Got it," I said.

"Really," she said again. "To their faces and when they're not around. We don't say mean things about our patients." I peered at her, in her cat-eye glasses, and wondered what I was missing.

They hired me for a six-month stint, likely because I speak Spanish. The afternoon I was hired, one of the other gals working there drove me down to Goodwill to pick out some secondhand scrubs. So I was official: a clinical person for the very first time.

Inside, the clinic looked like any other: a large waiting room, white hallways, an office with telephones. The only differences were that there were lamp-lit counseling spaces and each room was named after a famous woman. Indira Gandhi was the bathroom, until an Indian American patient pointed out that decorating a bathroom with a picture of Lakshmi, who is a god, could be insulting.

The clinic runs on antihierarchical principles. It is woman owned and woman run, and every person who works there trains in every position that interests her. Every other Saturday there were meetings for the entire staff, where we could bring up and discuss relevant issues. The only people who didn't come to these meetings were the doctors, because they didn't live in Austin. The doctors were scattered all over the state, and would fly in to Austin one or two days a week to provide abortions. Providing abortions in the same town where you live, I learned, can be dangerous. Also, many providers are family practitioners who don't want their primary care practices threatened by protestors.

I started out in the front office, which is the best place to learn how the clinic works. We in the front office were the first point of contact for women who needed an abortion. I answered the telephone. "So, I think I'm pregnant," the conversations would begin. Or just, "I'm pregnant." I took all the Spanish-speaking phone calls, because the senior gal in the office didn't speak Spanish. (I had learned to speak Spanish because the Port Aransas Rotary Club sent me off to be an exchange student in Spain my senior year of high school.) Sometimes, the women on the other end of the phone would whisper, or their voices would echo as if they were calling from behind a locked bathroom door. I learned to echo their feelings—*It can be a really scary thing*—and to gauge the term of the pregnancy from their last period. Most were in the first month of pregnancy. When they were ready to make an appointment, I would tell them what to expect.

First off, to comply with a Texas law requiring a mandatory

twenty-four-hour waiting period for women to get an abortion, our patients had to call a day before their appointment to listen to a recorded message about abortion. Not all the information in this message was true. The state had mandated that the message use the term "unborn child" rather than "fetus," and that women be told that abortion increases their risk of getting breast cancer. (It doesn't.) On the morning of the appointment, women would come in to start the complicated process of getting this simple procedure. First, they would get blood tests. That was followed by an ultrasound to verify the length of the pregnancy, and then (state-mandated) counseling by one of the clinic staff.

Women who were less than nine weeks pregnant could get a medical abortion, where they take medications that cause the fetus to detach from the uterus and the uterus to cramp—essentially inducing a miscarriage. The medical abortion could be done at home, after the women saw a doctor in the clinic. If the pregnancy was farther along or they felt safer doing it in the clinic, then we'd set them up for a surgical abortion, where the fetus is removed with suction. Rarely, pregnancies were advanced beyond sixteen weeks. In those cases, we would have to do a two-day procedure where dilators are placed into the cervix, and then left overnight before the abortion was done the next day.

Working in the front office, I was also trained on how to respond to a bomb threat. You alert someone to call the police, and try to get details about the bomb. A bomb threat never came while I was there.

"We're not Planned Parenthood," my boss explained, "so we don't get as many protestors."

I also learned how to answer women's questions.

Will it hurt? Yes, there is cramping-type pain, like you get with menstrual cramps, but more intense. We'll give you medication to control the pain.

Can I bring my sister? Yes.

What does the baby look like now?

I learned to answer that final question when I moved from the front office to the pathology lab. In the pathology lab, I had two jobs. First, I would clean and sterilize surgical instruments. But also, I would check the bottles that came back from the procedure room, to make sure that each contained the expected parts—amniotic sac, umbilical cord, fetus. I would pour the bottles over a strainer, rinse the blood away, and look. If anything was missing, the procedure might have to be repeated.

The pathology lab is where things grew more complicated for me. At the front office I had learned to describe how abortion works in appropriate, neutral terms. But in the pathology lab, I learned what the fetuses looked like.

The very early ones were soft and delicate. You could see the amniotic sac, which looked like a jellyfish, and the thin twisty umbilical cord that had connected it to the woman's bloodstream. There was no body. Many of the ones I saw were like this.

In later pregnancies, the fetuses were farther along, and they looked like little fish-people, with curved spines and tiny arms and legs. Some, more developed, just looked like the tiniest possible babies, but thin and red-skinned and bloody. My mind went cool and silent when I saw them, and I turned to my work with calm remove.

Everyone who worked at the clinic had abortion dreams, and mine began when I worked in the pathology lab. In the dream I would be driving, and the road was blocked by bloody bottles of tissue suctioned from inside a woman's body. Or I would be in the grocery store, and the fruit would be covered in slippery amniotic sacs. Another woman dreamed of performing an abortion on herself; yet another dreamed of a full-size baby emerging from a vagina and turning its head to stare at her. And so if we did our daily work as calm and warm professionals, the moral ambiguity emerged in dreams.

Despite the dreams, neither the pathology lab nor the front office changed my life. That came from counseling.

The state of Texas had mandated that every woman receive counseling before an abortion, and although the law was surely an attempt to add cost to care—bolstered by the patronizing notion that women couldn't make this decision on their own—we tried to use it for good. Counseling was the last step before the procedure. Alone with the patient in a private room, I would make sure all questions were answered and screen for women who were being coerced into having the abortion. But my real job was to support these women, and to listen to their stories.

Sometimes the women did not need to talk much. They just wanted their basic questions answered, and to get on with it. These were often women like me—white, college educated, blessed by a circle of supportive friends. But I also saw women who were living on the margins, and my Spanish-speaking women were more likely to come into the clinic with stories they had no other place to tell.

I know now that neither education nor friendship nor whiteness can spare us from the worst of the suffering that women go through. But at that time, it seemed to happen in this way. These stories, the stories that changed my life, were told in Spanish.

THE FIRST WAS NAYELI, whom I saw shortly after I had completed my counselor training and begun counseling patients on my own. She was sitting in the waiting room on a busy Saturday, clutching her bag—surrounded by other women, but alone. I called her back to the counseling room.

"Are you here by yourself?" I asked, opening the door to the lamp-lit counseling room.

"Yes, I couldn't tell anyone," she said.

"I'm so sorry, that must be hard." We sat down in the chairs, so close our knees could have touched. I quickly checked her chart to make sure she wasn't set up for IV pain control—no. She'd be able to drive herself home.

"Well, I have three kids, you know. And my sister is in Mexico. She would not understand. And my husband. No."

"No?" I asked.

"No," she said. "He does not, he would not understand this. If

he knew, he would suffer." I imagined her arriving home from her
abortion, breezing in the door with a forced smile, beginning dinner.

"Do you want to tell me about it?" I said.

She spoke quickly, words tumbling out to form the story that she
had not been able to tell to anyone else. "I did not want to get pregnant, you understand. But he, he won't use the condom. He will not
do it. I cannot make him do it."

"Okay," I said. "Okay. If you want to try the pill or something, we
can start you on that at your follow-up appointment."

"Yes," she said.

"So. How did you find out you were pregnant?"

"Well, I have three kids, so it was obvious," she said, spreading
her hands in the air before her belly. She was only a few weeks along.
"But now, but now. What will happen to me?" and she began crying.

"You're going to be okay," I said.

"No, I am not," she said. "It's—you don't understand. I'm Catholic."

"A lot of Catholic women come here," I said.

"I know. Oh, I know. And I have been praying and praying, but
there is no other way. I have to do it. My husband, he is a good man
and he works so hard. But there is no money, barely any money, not
enough. So I can barely feed my kids. My husband goes to bed hungry, you know, so that I can eat. And some days my children, they go
to bed hungry. And they are so small, you know, they don't understand about money. But they understand about hunger. It breaks my
heart."

"It breaks your heart," I said, simply repeating quietly what she
said to give her more space to talk.

"It breaks my heart, and if there were a fourth one, no. I cannot do
it. I have those three, and I have to feed them, and it is already more
than I can do."

"I understand," I said.

"You do, okay, but him!" and she pointed up, to the ceiling of the
clinic, beyond which stretched the branches of the live oaks and the
open sky. "God. God does not understand."

"God understands your heart in every moment," I said, grasping for some intuition of Catholicism that I did not really possess. "He knows you're acting out of love for your children."

And then the air seemed to grow perfectly still, because she stopped crying and looked straight at me and said quietly and firmly, "Yes. For them, I will go to hell."

THE SECOND STORY that changed my life was Gloria's. She was already in the counseling room when I went to meet her, because she had needed assistance to get there. She smiled from the chair where she was sitting, with her bandaged leg propped on a stool in front of her and her crutches leaning on the wall.

"I'm Rachel," I said, "your counselor."

"Hello," she said as I sat near her, and took my hand in both of hers. Kindness radiated into me from her. "Thank you."

"Oh, thank you," I said. And I began my spiel. "I'm here to explain the procedure, and to answer any questions you have, and also just to listen."

She nodded, and I went briefly through what would happen in the procedure room, finishing with "And then you'll rest up in the recovery room for as long as you need, and have a snack, and you can go when you're ready."

"Back to the shelter," she said. I nodded.

"And will I have a chance to say good-bye to my baby?" she asked.

"We could say good-bye together now, if you want," I said.

"I mean, could I see him? Could I see the baby afterwards?"

I thought of the slippery fetuses in the pathology room, and wondered what this kind woman would feel looking down at hers. She was eight weeks along, just far enough that there would be a little form along with the amniotic sac.

"If you want to," I said. "Of course you can."

"Everyone has been so kind to me," she said.

"Oh," I said. "Good."

"I mean," she said, laughing. "Except my husband."

I was so surprised by her laughter that I laughed, too.

"Can I show you?" she asked.

I paused. "Yes," I said, slowly. "If you want to."

"I want you to see," she said, "why I'm doing this." She leaned forward and pulled down the bandages over her thigh, and I saw the edge of the wound. Thick black stitches tracked down from the top of her thigh. "It goes from here," she said, "to here." And she traced the length of her thigh almost to the kneecap. "He wanted to kill me. I passed out from the blood loss, but the neighbors had heard me screaming and they called the police."

"My god," I said.

"I know he was trying to kill me," she said. "He slammed my head on the ground."

"I am so sorry."

"I love this baby, and I will not let it be born to him. This baby's life, and my life, would be tied to him forever."

"I understand," I said, my voice moving thinly through the air.

Later, I walked with her into the room where what remained of the body of her baby, the baby she loved, was waiting in a smooth glass bowl.

When I turned to leave her alone for a moment, I heard her begin to pray.

THE THIRD STORY that changed my life that year was Xochitl's. Xochitl was born in a Nahuatl village in Mexico, and when she was four years old her parents sold her.

"They sold you?" I asked, thinking surely I had misunderstood.

"Yes," she repeated. "They couldn't feed me, so they sold me. I went to work in a big ranch house, and I stayed there until I was sixteen and I ran away."

"Whoa," I said.

"Yes. I worked so hard." She took my hand in hers. "Feel my hands. I will never have soft, pretty hands like yours. I have been working as hard as I could since I was four years old." Her hands were small, and the skin was rough. When I touched them I could sense the truth of everything that I had heard. She was sitting face-to-face with me in the clinic and touching my hand. *She lives here,* I thought. *I might've passed her in the grocery store, and I would never know.*

"And the pregnancy?" I asked.

"Well, I am twenty-two now. And I do want to have babies," she said slowly. Then she leaned toward me, and brightened. "But listen to this," she said. "When I got pregnant, I realized that my boyfriend is a bastard! He steals my money, and he won't let me call my friends. I don't want to have his baby!"

"So this is a good choice for you," I said.

"Yes," she said firmly. "I have been through so much. But I have a job now. I make my own money. I have a place to live. I don't have to do what he tells me to do."

"So you're leaving him?" I asked.

"I already left him. That was the first real decision I ever made for myself, and this is the second," she said. "The abortion."

"You seem like a really strong person," I said.

"Maybe so," she said. "Somehow when I got pregnant, I realized that I was in a trap. But here is the miracle: I can get out."

THAT WORK IN THE CLINIC was the beginning of my life becoming unspeakable. So many of my stories are hard to tell. One does not go to a party and tell stories that end in "But the baby died three days later, with sepsis," or "And then we removed the old man's leg." One does not go to a party and speak of blood slipping down the drain at an abortion clinic. No story I could tell seemed like it would do justice to the women I had met, anyway, and so I began to keep a kind of silence that has become part of my professional life. I kept my old life up for a while, bicycling around my city, dancing, but it began to feel less and less real. I could not draw a thread between the life I lived outside of the clinic and the stories I heard there.

I left that job at the end of the summer and, as I had planned before I got the job at the clinic, I moved to New York. If my life in Austin had felt unreal, New York was hyperreal, and I was outside of it the whole time. I would go to writing workshops in the MFA program I had enrolled in at Columbia, and care, passionately but briefly, about the stories we were telling. When a friend got pregnant I thought, *Mothering is a sacred thing. Did you know that I met a mother who gave up her immortal soul in order to feed her children?* But I didn't say it. I said congratulations, as you do. Women I knew fell in love with men, and I thought, *He seems like a wonderful man. But sometimes they try to kill you,* my mind tracing the stitches up and down Gloria's thigh. She would be walking again now; she would have a scar.

The public debate about abortion rights hummed on and sometimes flared, and always seemed to have little to do with either the fetuses—those slippery little almost-lives, those bodies I myself could not look at for long—or the women. It seemed mostly about male politicians and abstract morality. Certainly no political discussion could hold half of Xochitl's strength, Gloria's kindness, or Nayeli's determination. As I drifted through my unreal life and a pretty fall turned into a biting, big-city winter, my mind continued wandering back to the clinic. The counseling room had felt sacred to me: there, women shared stories that could be told in no other place. I remembered the touch of Xochitl's rough hands, and how instantly I had recognized her story as true. That space, the clinic room, was real.

One night I sat on a bench overlooking Morningside Park, taking sips of tequila from a flask with a friend who was also a writer in the master's program. She too felt uneasy in New York.

"I think about dropping out of the program all the time," I said.

"So do I," she said. "But I don't know what else I'd do. I've always been a writer."

"Sure," I said.

From the bench, we could see down over the tops of the trees in the park, and the lights of Harlem stretching away on the other side.

"What would you do?" she asked.

"I'd go to medical school," I said without hesitating. As I spoke, the plan began to take shape. I wanted to be back in the clinic, back in that storytelling space—but more than that, I wanted my life to feel solid again. I wanted to work all day, and see what I had done at the end of the day. I wanted to be useful.

"Well," my friend said. "That makes sense."

CHAPTER 3

I LEFT THE WRITING PROGRAM IN DECEMBER OF 2006, and the next step on my path toward medical school took me to Portland, Oregon, for a "postbac," a postbaccalaureate premedical program. These programs are designed for the truly masochistic student who wishes to complete all of her premed classes—general chemistry, organic chemistry, physics, calculus, and biology—in a single year. I found a room on Craigslist in early June, and my parents drove me across the country to drop me off.

Portland is the kind of liberal town where a lesbian friend of mine could decide to recycle the double-ended dildo that she and her partner were bored with, and the city workers would haul it away without comment. There were dead volcanoes within the city limits, and so many waterfalls nearby that I felt a bit oppressed. ("Texas has a subtle beauty," I said once, dismissing a sixty-foot waterfall with a wave of my hand. "It's not all flashy and in-your-face.") I got a red bicycle, named it "Squeaky," and memorized the periodic table. Flowers bloomed all summer: poppies in the neighbors' yard, passionflowers climbing up the fences I passed on my way to the library.

My house was a little safe haven on the southeast side, full of young people who had just moved to Portland. There was Corey, the landlord, a photographer who also worked on a commercial crab boat. There was Sara, the beautiful Australian (favorite animal: wombat), and Heather, a really decent human being who counseled college students. Heather had a genetically deficient white cat named Brian, who liked to defecate on white things (carpet, comforters, paper). Once, Brian got stuck in a tree just four feet off the ground, and we all gathered in the yard to mock him.

I felt happy at home, but I was lonely at school. It was my own fault: I had convinced myself that I was a "writer"—a very different sort of creature from the average premed student. These other pre-meds were squares who seemed to wear only rain gear. The vaunted fashion and coolness of Portland was not on display in the General Chemistry course at Portland State.

To be honest, my sense of superiority came from fear. I feared that all these other people, these squares, were right for medicine, whereas I myself could never be a good doctor—not with my liberal arts degree, my wandering mind, and my dark sense of humor. *I'm too cool for this,* I told myself, when really I was afraid I wasn't good enough. So I sat by myself in class and stewed over the elements, until the day I sat down next to Frank.

I was late to class, holding a cup of coffee and sloughing rain off the sides of my gigantic brown jacket. Hoping to go unnoticed by our chemistry professor, I snuck in a side door. But all the rows were filled. I clumped and dripped up the stairs, feeling increasingly exposed, until someone hissed, "Here. You can sit down here."

That someone was a thin young man with curly blond hair and a huge smile. "Thank god," I whispered to him. "I'm terrified of all these people."

"Me too!" he whispered, and patted my arm.

Frank and I recognized each other instantly. We were both in a sort of hiding, assuming that our true selves could never get into medical school. He—for the first time since junior high—was trying to hide the fact that he was gay. Our ideas about doctors were mostly unfounded, because neither of us had had regular medical care growing up, but we took doctors seriously. Doctors, we figured, were straight white men. They were rational creatures, content to spend a thousand sunny afternoons in the laboratory macerating rat lungs to extract a protein. They were calm, and a bit humorless.

Frank and I were not like that. We laughed our way through general chemistry, which—to our mutual shock—we aced. "We understand science!" we squealed when we got our grades.

We also laughed about our families. I showed him a picture of myself with my crooked teeth in the trailer park days, and told him the story of the time my cousin divorced her husband without telling him about it. ("That's so trashy!" he whispered with delight. "Exactly!" I said.) At the end of the summer, Frank went on a weekend trip to the lake with his family, which he chronicled for me in hilarious detail: with his latest stepfather, his mother, and a set of cousins, he had stayed in a cabin on the lake. His grandmother Ma, who was the most stable and loving person in Frank's life, had not attended. One day the family went tubing, pulling ski tubes behind a boat. The trip had taken a year to save up for, but Frank's mom was pretty stressed the whole time. At one point she fell off the dock. He said I was the only person who could laugh so hard with him at something that was actually so sad.

As summer cooled into fall, Frank and I became lab partners in every class and study buddies every night. Frank knitted quietly beside me through three lectures about the reptile kidney; I wrote a poem for *Rattus norvegicus* and marveled at the perceptive powers of the pit viper. (Those pits on their skulls sense infrared radiation from the warm bodies of mice, but neuroscience has shown that the viper experiences the heat as an image—like what we would see with our eyes!) In lab, we explored the electrical properties of the zebrafish, used simple machines, and transformed acids into salts. "Voilà!" Frank would say, waving his hand over a beaker. "Science!"

It never stopped feeling like a miracle that Frank and I could do well in science classes. Yet we did, and mostly because we studied fanatically, together. As I became closer with Frank, I began to drop the idea that I was too cool to be a regular premed. Our giant text-books became a badge of honor, which we would proudly lug from place to place. We were a comfort to each other: If Frank could make it in medicine, so could I. If medicine could be a place where we would meet the true friends of our hearts, then maybe we both were going to be okay.

Between problem sets, we would analyze each other's relationships with men. Frank desperately wanted to be in love, whereas I had an abundance of love but no real sense of direction with relationships.

"Why would you kiss him?" he squealed when I told him I had kissed a random guy whom I didn't think was very smart.

"I honestly don't know," I said, and he looked at me with wonder. From Frank's perspective, a straight woman who had an easy chance to find real love, but seemed instead to wander through meaningless encounters, was wasting the chance he desperately wanted for him-self. Sometimes he would do the math: If 10 percent of people were gay and half of those were men, and 20 percent of those were in his age range, then he could potentially find love with one in every one hundred people. That meant 1 percent of the Portland population, or, as he would put it brightly, "Nearly six thousand potential boyfriends right here in the City of Roses!"

But in our premed classes—the community where we spent most of our waking time—the chances felt slimmer. The anxiety of apply-ing to medical school, and trying to conform to some notion of the archetypal good doctor, worked its way into Frank. Although nobody in our community was mean to Frank, and nobody told him that a gay man can't be a doctor, Frank had gotten a subtle message—just as I had—that a doctor is a certain kind of person. "I worry about it," he told me. "How will I hide it in interviews?"

"Do you have to hide it?" I asked him.

"Yes," he said. And I figured he knew more about the subject than I did. Frank didn't come out to most people in class; he didn't brighten up and laugh hysterically at my dumb jokes until we were well away from campus.

Nor did the gay community, which Frank had been a vibrant part of during his college days in Eugene, feel like a safe haven to him. "Sometimes I think the gay community here is pathological," he said with sadness. "We all just got so messed up in high school. We were really taught to hate ourselves. And then you're supposed to just be able to open up and love someone who symbolizes everything you hate about yourself."

As the rainy fall progressed to the dark and rainy winter, Frank and I moved from being study friends to being real friends. There was a stand of bright yellow trees in a park downtown that he loved; they kept their color until November. After class we'd walk arm in arm under those yellow trees to Powell's Books, where I started reading poetry and Frank taught me what brioche was. On Sundays, he would come over for dinner. He was having a hard time eating that winter, but he loved the fish tacos I made from halibut that my brother sent from Alaska. I would send Frank home with a Tupperware container full of fish.

But by January, the rain was getting me down. The rain, the darkness, and studying for the MCAT. Why does anybody ever leave the great state of Texas, where winters are sunny?

"Rain makes the flowers grow!" Frank said. So I nicknamed him "Cloudforest."

"Cloudforest," I would say, "we understand physics."

One Thursday afternoon, Frank and I sat on a couch at our usual coffee shop to do organic chemistry homework. I was complaining about a new housemate—Ron, who washed his whole body twice a day with antibacterial soap and had screamed at me twice for touching his dishes. Frank suggested that we use science to "take him out," and we giggled over the idea, then got very nerdy. We were in the middle of a three-day experiment in organic chemistry lab, distilling caffeine from tea. "Could you use caffeine?" Frank asked.

We figured that you could. We figured caffeine could kill a pesky roommate, and probably by arrhythmia. Then we talked about other things. Frank was worried about passing the MCAT. My grand-mother had paid for me to take an MCAT prep course, but Frank had no such help. He told me that he was down, really down. He was doing all the right things to try and feel better—exercise, knitting, seeing his counselor. He'd gone on an antidepressant. But nothing was helping. We talked a while, just so close on that couch that our forearms were brushing, then walked down to the bookstore. I met another friend there, and Frank and I said good-bye. He was never very much for mixing friend groups, having long cultivated a habit of keeping parts of his own life secret.

That Sunday night, I didn't call Frank and he did not call me. It was the first time in months we hadn't had Sunday dinner.

FRANK WAS MISSING ON MONDAY. In eight a.m. biology he missed a quiz, which was totally unlike him. I called, and left a mes-sage. *Cloudforest, this is Rachel. You missed a quiz! I'm worried about you; call me back.*

I was worried enough that our friend Amy drove me over to Frank's house to look for him between classes. The door was locked. There was a pecan tree in the yard, and I threw fallen pecans at his window. It was February, and they were soft with rot. The pecans tapped against Frank's window, but he did not respond.

Amy drove me back to campus for organic chemistry class, where Frank missed a test. Impossible. He was ranked third in our class in organic chemistry, and proud of it. He didn't miss tests. After the test, I bicycled home. I looked up Frank's housemate Dean on the Internet, and called him at work asking him to go home and check on Frank. He agreed. He would go straight home.

Then time began to move very slowly.

I sat in the window seat of my bedroom, watching the wind trou-ble some leaves on the asphalt far below. I don't know how long I sat there, but finally I realized that Dean had not called back.

———

WHEN I ARRIVED at Frank's house, the medical examiner's truck was parked outside. The front door was open, and I walked in to find Dean and a man in police uniform and a woman in a dress standing silently in the foyer.

"No," I said.

"Rachel," Dean said. I had never met him before.

"Frank?" I asked.

"I'm so sorry," Dean said, and he stepped toward me and hugged me hard for a long time. So without anybody saying it, I knew that Frank was dead.

"When you called," Dean said, "I didn't expect. I didn't know that he would be there in his room." So Dean had been asleep in the next room while Frank quietly killed himself, and then came home to find his housemate dead in his bed.

"Oh my god, I'm so sorry," I said.

"I didn't know," he repeated.

"Of course not," I said.

"Do you want . . . do you want to sit?" he said. So I sat down on the couch next to the strange woman, who introduced herself as a social worker, and the three of us waited while the medical examiner went upstairs and came back again.

"There's a note," he said when he returned. "Do you want to read it?"

Dean said no, he didn't think he could handle it right then, but I said yes.

In the note, Frank described how he killed himself with caffeine. He had gone out in the style of a good science student: well researched, precise, effective, using a simple method we had studied in organic chemistry lab. He even described researching the lethal dose.

Frank wrote that he had thought about suicide for a long time. He used to think about throwing himself off of one of Portland's bridges, but he didn't want his body to be all waterlogged. (I remembered saying good-bye to him on a bridge one night, how he waved hugely and bounced away toward home with his book bag. He did not seem preoccupied with the water, then.)

Frank signed the note, "I love you, Mom and Ma." His mother and his grandmother, who did not yet know that he was dead. Would police be headed toward their home right now?

My name and phone number, along with those of two other friends, were written on the bottom of the note. Frank, so conscientious, knew we would inform anybody who needed to know.

I didn't go to look at his body, but the medical examiner told me about the room. There were NoDoz scattered on the carpet, and the Wikipedia page for caffeine was open on his computer. A Tupperware container of fish that I'd cooked—maybe his dinner, or maybe meant for lunch the next day?—was on his bedside table.

FOR A FEW DAYS, I was dysfunctional with grief. Some people brought food, and eventually I ate. So many people called with condolences that, in a moment of exhaustion, I dropped my ringing telephone into a glass of water beside my bed. It was a relief.

My new housemate John Johnson drove me from place to place, held me while I wept, and stayed up nights playing board games or watching *Saturday Night Live* reruns with me—anything to turn my mind from the loss. When I slept, I dreamed that I was hanging out with Frank. In the dream I said, "I'm so relieved! I thought that you were dead!" and Frank laughed and shook his head no. Then I woke up and began sobbing when I remembered what had happened.

I had a few rambling telephone conversations with Frank's mother, who called to thank me for being Frank's friend after finding my number on the suicide note. She asked me to bring Frank's favorite sweater home for him to be cremated in, and John was ready to drive me across the state until she called again and changed her mind. People moved around me gently, saying that I should take all the time I needed. If I needed to drop some classes, or leave school for a while, I should. "Medical school's not going anywhere," they said.

And so, for a few days, I stayed home. *Who would I sit next to in class?* I wondered. *Who would be my lab partner?*

Then, later that week, my father called.

"I'm so sorry, kiddo," he began. We talked for a while, and then I told him that I was thinking of taking a break from school.

"I don't think that's a good idea," he said. And then he went on. "This is an awful thing. And it's the first time this has happened to you, sweetie. But you know what? It's not going to be the last."

I was silent. There was a firmness in his voice that I had not heard from anyone else that week.

"You know I dropped out of college," he said. "Well, I had started taking classes up there in Arkansas, and one day I got home and found that my friend had blown his brains out with a shotgun. And I left. I left, and I never made it back. And that wasn't the last time I lost someone like that. But you know what? You're not going to leave."

"Dad—" I began.

"No, listen to me now. I love you. And I know you. I probably know you better than anybody else knows you, because you're so much like me. I know who you come from. Your grandfather was a Marine. He fought on the Pacific front in World War II, and only 20 percent of his battalion survived. He saw all his friends get shot. Over and over. One of his best friends was shot in the face right next to him. And you know what, Rachel?"

"What?"

"Your granddad came home alive, and he was a happy guy. Listen, Rachel. He was a happy guy."

"Dad—"

"I'm not done. Your grandmother. She was diagnosed with cancer in her fifties, just a few years after she started teaching. And you know what she did?"

"What, Dad?" I asked quietly.

"She kept on teaching. She got that double mastectomy, and all that chemotherapy, and all that radiation, and she fought cancer for twenty years straight. She did not stop teaching. She woke up one morning and all her toenails had fallen out, and you know what she did?"

"What's that, Dad?"

"She put on her socks and her sandals and she went to work. So that's what you're going to do, kiddo. I know you. These are the people you come from, and this is who you are."

One should not count on a working-class father to soft pedal grief. He knew how much I was hurting, because he'd been through it, too. But he didn't stop expecting the greatest effort from me.

I did not drop out. I did not stop going to class. And even though for a long time I wondered if I had failed Frank by not walking the desert of grief for long enough in his honor, I have never forgotten my father's words. *These are the people you come from. This is who you are.*

FRANK'S FUNERAL was held the next weekend in his hometown. I drove over with our friend Michael, and there was snow on the mountain passes. We pulled up to the VFW in Michael's dark car, and found the funeral gathering in the fluorescent-lit meeting room, where photos of Frank were clustered at the front and the walls were decorated with the usual VFW regalia: war memorabilia, a poster board with community announcements, another with the twelve tenets of Alcoholics Anonymous. The crowd was varied: a few premeds, a group of devastated young men from Eugene, and then Frank's family. Several stepdads were there, in jeans and button-downs. Frank's mom wore a long black dress, and his beloved grandmother, who had been the rock of stability in his youth, held a calm face.

"You're Rachel," she said, when I introduced myself. "He loved you."

"You're Ma," I said. "He loved you so much. I'm sorry."

"It's an awful thing," she said.

I felt awkward about my own calm face, as others were weeping around me. "I'm sorry, I don't cry as much," I said. "I've been crying a lot at home."

"Don't worry, honey," she said. "People show their grief in different ways." And so, not for the last time, a person who was suffering more than I could know reached out to comfort me.

The funeral had been unexpected and hastily arranged, of course, but everyone did their best. Frank's mother had put together a heartbreaking slide show to begin the ceremony: baby pictures of Frank and childhood pictures, with two of Frank's favorite songs—one by Sarah McLachlan and one by Antony and the Johnsons. There was Frank graduating from high school, then college. There was Frank with the long blond curls he cut in order to look like a good premedical student. And there was the Frank I knew, twenty-six years old and alive, laughing broadly in his periodic-table-of-the-elements T-shirt.

The preacher who spoke did not know Frank, and he said as much, but he finished the ceremony by saying that Frank's mother wanted to add a message. The message was this: "I want everyone to know that Frank did not mean to leave us."

When I spoke with Frank's mom afterward, it became clear what her message meant: she knew that some antidepressants could increase the risk of suicide, and she wanted to sue the doctor who had prescribed them for Frank. "What do you think?" she asked me.

"I don't know," I said. "I guess I just don't know."

She was trying to make sense of the death, and I would see many people try to do the same at the various memorials I attended in Frank's name over the next week. Some said that he had killed himself because he was gay, and he was pushed into conformity by the premedical curriculum. Some blamed it on depression. Some quietly blamed his family; some blamed homophobic society. I never could make much sense of it myself. In my grief I refused all explanations, as if putting labels on Frank's life or his death would do violence to the complicated and beautiful person he was.

I did feel guilty, though. If my mind grasped at any easy explanation, it was, *This was your fault. You should've known. When he told you about the depression, when you joked about killing someone with caffeine. Those were messages, and you should have understood.*

If I had called him that Sunday night, maybe he wouldn't have made an impulsive decision. If I had loved Frank better, or shared the online exams from my MCAT prep course with him. My mind could twist any detail into a knot of blame.

Gradually, though, I healed. Healing meant accepting that Frank's death was not my fault. Maybe he had tried to reach out to me, and maybe I had missed it. Just as I was involved in his life—that Tupperware of fish at his bedside table, my phone number on the bottom of the note—I had been involved in his death. I was involved because we were truly friends, and we loved each other.

One night I dreamed that my brother and I were driving together through the darkness in the pickup truck that we shared in college. We arrived at the lake in Montgomery, and my brother slowly navigated the truck into the shallow water. The headlights played out over the water in the darkness, and my brother nodded silently to me. I pulled the door handle, and stepped out into the water. I leaned over and began searching through the water with my hands. I knew I was looking for a body, but I didn't know if I would find my own body, or Frank's. Finally I found him, thin and dripping and dead, and I lifted him gently from the water and placed him in the back of the truck. I got back in beside my brother, and we drove away.

CHAPTER 4

I INTERVIEWED FOR MEDICAL SCHOOL ALL OVER THE COUNTRY, but nothing out of Texas felt quite right.

At NYU, for example, all the medical students live in a tower directly above the medical school. "We elevator commute!" my tour guide announced jocularly. When I asked if any of the students refrained from living in the tower directly above the medical school, he scratched his head for a minute and said, "Well, there is one girl who lives in Brooklyn. But nobody really hangs out with her much. I think she has kids or something?"

The radiologist who interviewed me there also mentioned the tower. "Oh," she said. "That's exactly how you have to do it. You must," she said. "You must live in the tower directly above the medical school."

When I asked her if, as a radiologist, she missed interacting with patients, she said simply, "No."

I got wait-listed.

At another fancy school, I asked a student panel what percentage of graduates go into primary care.

"Oh, don't worry," a student answered solemnly. "If you come to school here, you don't *have* to go into primary care."

Afterward, another student—a woman—came up and grabbed my wrist. "Hey," she whispered.

"Um, hey," I said.

"Listen, I'm going into general pediatrics," she whispered.

"Okay," I whispered.

"I just wanted you to know," she whispered.

"Why are we whispering?" I whispered.

"I guess some people feel like it's a waste of my education," she said. "Like, if you go here, you should become a specialist."

After one particularly devastating interview in New York City, I called my friend Jonathan, in Chicago. All day I had been thinking of Frank: how much he would've loved to be in my place, touring the hospital in a brand-new suit. I felt the weight of going on, and going to medical school, without him. At that time I felt that he deserved it more, and that I had not mourned him enough. I had returned to classes too soon after his death.

Jonathan spoke slowly, his voice crackling over to me from Chicago. "If we mourned fully any one loss," he said, "that would take a whole lifetime."

He paused. "But other things happen."

ONE PLACE THAT DID FEEL RIGHT was the University of Texas Medical Branch (UTMB) on Galveston Island. On Galveston, I had a built-in group of friends who I knew through my friend Margaret, who was an MD/PhD student there. They all lived in a yellow Victorian house halfway between the medical school and the beach. After every test, my friend Katie would bicycle down to the water and throw herself in. Then she would bicycle home, rinse the sand from her feet with a garden hose, step inside, and fix herself a gin and tonic. That seemed, to me, like a livable life.

Margaret, Katie, and their friend Emily were all student directors at the St. Vincent's Student-Run Free Clinic, where eventually I would meet Mr. Rose. St. Vincent's—the clinic—is a medical clinic staffed by volunteer students and physicians from UTMB. The free clinic operates in collaboration with St. Vincent's House—the House—which is a historically black community center and an Episcopal mission house. The House is a hub of crucial services for working-class and poor Galvestonians. It has a school where people can get a GED or learn English, a food pantry, a chapel, and a pre-school. The House's second story holds eight exam rooms, which are shared by a nurse-managed day clinic and the student-run free clinic. The student-run clinic operates every Tuesday and Thursday evening, as well as Saturday during the day. The House provides the space, a paid receptionist, and office needs such as printers and Internet access. UTMB supports the clinic by paying for blood tests and Pap smears to be run, and the rest is paid for by grants (including some grants from UTMB), donations, and volunteer labor. The main annual fund-raiser is a talent show.

Twenty blocks east of St. Vincent's is the main UTMB campus, a large complex of buildings dedicated to research, education, and patient care. There are lecture halls and small-group rooms for the schools of medicine, nursing, and allied health professions, as well as for the Graduate School of Biological Sciences. There are massive laboratory buildings including the Galveston National Lab, a biosafety level-four facility that houses research on measles, Ebola, anthrax, and other highly infectious diseases. There is a hospital complex composed of four separate hospitals linked together. The main hospital is John Sealy, but there is also Rebecca Sealy, the nearby Shriners Burns Hospital, a children's hospital, and Hospital Galveston. Hospital Galveston is a maximum-security prison hospital where UTMB providers treat prisoners from across the state. Hospital Galveston is right on campus, linked to John Sealy Hospital by a sky bridge.

Galveston had the Institute for the Medical Humanities, where I could do a PhD that would bring together my interests in medicine and the arts. Galveston had a historic seawall built in 1901, an aquarium with a baby hammerhead shark, and a dive bar called the Poop Deck. And, for much of the last century, UTMB had been a flagship charity hospital serving poor and uninsured patients from across the state. The students I met at UTMB were mission oriented: they were proud to be part of a hospital with a long history of caring for the poor.

UTMB had already begun to cut back on charity care by the time I was applying. But there was no way to know, then, the full scope of what would happen. On September 13, 2008, just a week before my UTMB interview, I opened up my computer to find that Galveston was underwater.

TO UNDERSTAND GALVESTON you have to understand hurricanes. Barrier islands protect the mainland from these storms. When hurricanes hit, barrier islands like Galveston take the brunt of the storm's destructive force.

One hurricane, the Great Storm of 1900, had already changed the character of the island forever. Before the Great Storm, Galveston was the main port for the Southwestern United States. The Southern Pacific Railroad begins there, and the town boomed in the nineteenth century as cotton, wheat, and tobacco flowed through the port. Immigrants came, too: Galveston was the Ellis Island of the South. It was also a slave port until the federal order for emancipation arrived in Texas in 1865.* The party in the streets of Galveston on June 19, 1865, gave rise to the Juneteenth holiday celebrating the emancipation of American slaves. After emancipation, black civic leaders in Galveston established the state's first black high school and black public library. Statesman and former slave Norris Wright Cuney led black dockworkers to unionize and to campaign successfully for fair pay.

* Yup, 1865. Texas resisted emancipation from 1863 to 1865, and did not act on the new law until forced to do so.

Today, many Galvestonians are nostalgic for the 1890s, when our city was progressive and rich—a temperate barrier island of towering stone churches and cobbled streets, home of the state's first medical school. On September 8, 1900, that Galveston was utterly destroyed.

The Great Storm of 1900 killed six thousand people and wrecked nearly every structure on the island. The bridges to the mainland were knocked out, and the city was out of communication for days afterward, while newspapers around the world shared news of the storm. So many dead bodies were left in the wreckage that Galveston men were forced at bayonet-point to gather the bodies and load them onto barges for burial at sea. The men were given whiskey to help them cope with the awful stench. But the barge-loads of dumped bodies were carried back to the island on the waves, and finally, Galvestonians torched them in massive funeral pyres.

Reports from those who witnessed the Great Storm were surreal: One doctor wrote of coming across the corpse of a woman with "a half-born babe" protruding from her. Another described orgies in the streets of the devastated city—likely a tall tale. Cholera swept through. "The story of Galveston's tragedy," resident Ida Parker Austin wrote, "can never be written."

The story of Galveston itself could have ended then. But 1900 was a time of progress in America, and Texans were a hardy lot. Like their descendants who would respond to the Great Depression of the 1930s with a massive public works investment, Galvestonians responded to the Great Storm by rebuilding—and building better. The U.S. Army Corps of Engineers was brought in to construct a seawall on the ocean-facing south side of Galveston. This eighteen-foot-high seawall would protect the island from the battering waves of any future hurricane, but it meant that the grade of the entire island would have to be raised. And so Galvestonians spent six years walking from house to house on wooden catwalks, while remaining structures were winched up from the earth, and silt from the bay was pumped in to form new, higher ground under the island. Today, the island still slopes gradually down from eighteen feet above sea level at the seawall, to just above sea level at Broadway, then to the level of the bay on the north side of the island.

On New Year's Day 1901, the Galveston *Daily News* ran a story covering the damage from the Great Storm and the construction and repair that was already well under way. The headline read, GALVESTON WAS NOT BORN TO DIE!

Galveston survived, but it never again was the promising major city it had been. The live oaks on the island were replanted by the Women's Public Health Association and, for a century, the seawall worked.

It didn't work for everybody, however. When Galveston was forcibly segregated, the seawall defined the geography of segregation. Black families were restricted to the low-lying north side of the island, beyond where the grade had been raised. The north side would be home to African American neighborhoods throughout the twentieth century, as black communities took root there.

Other hurricanes came and went after 1900, leaving the south side intact. The north side of the island, including the downtown and the port area, flooded again in 1915 and then again with Hurricane Carla in 1961. The Galvestonians of the north side rebuilt.

Then came Hurricane Rita. In 2005, three weeks after Hurricane Katrina devastated New Orleans, Galvestonians went through a tedious and costly evacuation—including the first-ever total evacuation of John Sealy Hospital—for Rita. Hundreds of UTMB patients were evacuated by helicopter or ambulance. Katrina and the ghastly events at storm-bound Memorial Medical Center in New Orleans were certainly on the minds of the UTMB officials who opted for a total evacuation for Rita.* The 2005 evacuation cost UTMB $25 million, and that loss coincided with a $50 million cut to the university's budget from the state legislature. This coincidence of budget cuts and a costly evacuation is one early root of the troubles that

---

* Karen Sexton, Lynn Alperin, and John Stobo, "Lessons from Hurricane Rita: The University of Texas Medical Branch Hospital's Evacuation," *Academic Medicine* 82, no. 8 (August 2007): 792–796.

would lead UTMB to abandon its historical mission as a charity care hospital.

With most everyone from Galveston, Houston, and the surrounding towns suddenly on the roads, the evacuation for Hurricane Rita was the largest single mass movement of Americans since the Dust Bowl. But Rita turned. It hit a less populated area of the coast at the Louisiana border, sparing Galveston and Houston. More Gulf Coast residents died from heat and exhaustion during the massive evacuation than were killed by Hurricane Rita itself.

Then in 2008, the year I was applying to medical school, came Hurricane Ike.

ON THE MORNING OF SEPTEMBER 11, 2008, Hurricane Ike made a sharp turn toward Galveston Island. The National Weather Service report at 4:19 p.m. read:

LIFE-THREATENING INUNDATION LIKELY!

ALL NEIGHBORHOODS . . . AND POSSIBLY ENTIRE
COASTAL COMMUNITIES . . . WILL BE INUNDATED
DURING THE PERIOD OF PEAK STORM TIDE. PERSONS
NOT HEEDING EVACUATION ORDERS IN SINGLE-
FAMILY ONE- OR TWO-STORY HOMES WILL FACE
CERTAIN DEATH. MANY RESIDENCES OF AVERAGE
CONSTRUCTION DIRECTLY ON THE COAST WILL
BE DESTROYED. WIDESPREAD AND DEVASTATING
PERSONAL PROPERTY DAMAGE IS LIKELY ELSEWHERE.
VEHICLES LEFT BEHIND WILL LIKELY BE SWEPT AWAY.
NUMEROUS ROADS WILL BE SWAMPED . . . SOME MAY BE
WASHED AWAY BY THE WATER. ENTIRE FLOOD PRONE
COASTAL COMMUNITIES WILL BE CUT OFF. WATER
LEVELS MAY EXCEED NINE FEET FOR MORE THAN A
MILE INLAND . . .

———

ACROSS THE ISLAND and in the little towns around it, St. Vincent's patients—and nearly everyone else—scrambled to evacuate. Vanessa, a patient in her fifties who lived just off the island, figured that she and her husband Jimmy would escape the worst of it. She was grateful that she didn't have her kids or grandkids with her when the hurricane came. It meant that all she had to deal with was herself, Jimmy, and the animals.

The animals included a battered Chihuahua that Vanessa had nursed back to health, a sad-faced pit bull she found abandoned by the highway, and a formerly abused macaw that would greet Jimmy every evening when he came home from work at the refinery. There were two baby squirrels she found near death after their mother was run over on the highway, a rabbit, and more dogs.

"I wasn't going to leave my animals behind!" Vanessa told me later. "You never know how long it's going to take before they let you come back, and you may not have power or nothing for weeks." To evacuate all these animals, Jimmy hooked a trailer to the back of their pickup, and they loaded up crates and cages, and headed north. The macaw rode up front in the cab.

With a mandatory evacuation in effect all along the coast, the drive up to central Texas took nearly sixteen hours. Rain battered the truck. There were hours-long lines at gas stations. Emergency shelters were open in Houston, but Vanessa didn't want to go to a shelter, where she'd be separated from her animals. Then again, there was no money for a hotel, not with what they were putting into gas. Vanessa had been out of work since a car wreck the year before messed up her back, so Jimmy's salary was all they had.

They crept north through the heavy evacuation traffic until they hit a state park in central Texas. But they were turned away there—too many animals. As they were leaving the park, Vanessa heard a strange noise from the trailer. She went back to check the animals, and a puppy was having a seizure. "That near broke my heart," Vanessa said.

She and Jimmy drove to an emergency vet, where the puppy was treated for low blood sugar. And the veterinarian, seeing how exhausted Vanessa and Jimmy looked, said they could camp in the parking lot. Vanessa wept with relief. And there they stayed, walking the animals on leashes, until it was safe to go back toward Galveston.

The TV in the vet's office rolled coverage of Ike. The flooding was awful. Nineteen people were dead. Somebody's pet tiger escaped after the storm and was roaming the Bolivar Peninsula. The hurricane passed over central Texas on Saturday, but the worst brute force of the winds and rain had gone.

MEDICAL STUDENT KRISTY MITCHELL did not plan to evacuate. She owned her home, because Galveston is the kind of decayed glorious city where a medical student can buy a house with a turret and finance it partly on student loans. She was a St. Vincent's director, and a fourth-year student with strong ties to the island. When the National Guard knocked on her door the day before the storm, Kristy was baking popovers.

Kristy evacuated, but nearly one-third of Galvestonians did not. A whole contingent of Galvestonians decided to ride out the storm at the Poop Deck, which was right on the seawall. Ike was only a Category 2 storm—it didn't sound so bad.

Hurricanes are categorized according to wind speed. As a Category 2, Ike had winds of up to 110 miles per hour. What made Ike so devastating was not merely strong winds, but the size of the hurricane. Nearly six hundred miles across, it covered much of the Gulf of Mexico and caused a massive storm surge before it. This storm surge sank Galveston: The seawall protected buildings on the north side of the island, but the storm surge pushed water into the bay, flooding the island from behind. Just as in 1915 and 1961, the north side of the island got the worst of it. The flood knocked out the whole first floor of St. Vincent's House, where the preschool had been. The clinic areas on the upper story were spared.

"Everybody knew this neighborhood would flood," Michael Thomas Jackson, the minister of St. Vincent's House, said to me. "We're sitting here at three feet below sea level." As went New Orleans, so went Galveston: The black community, having once been segregated to flood-prone neighborhoods, remained there. They put down roots—or they were unable to escape—until they were forced out after the hurricane.

KRISTY'S ROOMMATE RIMMA snuck back onto the island the week after Ike hit, flashing a UTMB badge to get past three checkpoints where National Guardsmen with huge guns strapped to their chests shifted and stared on the causeway leading to the island. "I just said, 'We're with UTMB,'" Rimma said. She did not say that she was a first-year medical student.

The people who had been living in Galveston's public housing did not get back so easily. Many were bussed to shelters across the state. When the buses attempted to return, they were sent back at the checkpoint—the "look-and-leave" policy for Galveston residents that had been enacted a week after the storm was abruptly canceled. When people tried again to return, many learned that they had no homes to return to. The public housing, home to about six thousand Galvestonians, was all condemned. St. Vincent's was not condemned, nor were many of the flooded buildings on the north side. Debate would rage for years over exactly why the public housing was condemned instead of repaired, with many people seeing it as a deliberate move to force out the poor. And Galveston would drag its feet rebuilding the public housing, delaying even after the federal government ordered the city to rebuild. In the meantime, the people who used to live there—including many people who loved Galveston, and had generations of family in town—scattered across the state and beyond.

Passing the guardsmen, Rimma saw wrecked boats cast adrift on the road, broken lumber and shingles, miles of wreckage strewn over the east end of Galveston. The fetid water had receded, leaving a thick layer of sludge laced with pollutants, including arsenic and lead from the flooded refineries in Galveston and Texas City.

UTMB is also north of Broadway, and so the first floor of most buildings was flooded. Critical hospital employees—enough to run a streamlined emergency room and operating room if the need should arise—had stayed through the storm. The hospital power failed because the generators were in the flooded basement, and so the docs and nurses spent the day of the storm in darkness, listening to wind and rain batter the hospital. When a technician managed to rig up enough power to turn on the red-and-blue UTMB light atop the hospital tower, everybody cheered. The light sent a bright signal across the devastated island: the hospital was open.

One UTMB building spared from flooding was the Galveston National Lab. The lab had been built to be hurricane-proof, so there were only two signs of damage there. At the first-floor entrance, a welcome carpet was damp. And hundreds of research animals had to be killed when backup power failed.

In the days after the storm, power was routed to essential buildings where patient care and temperature-sensitive research was going on. Elsewhere, the power (including the air-conditioning) was cut. In the UTMB anatomy lab, the human cadavers that first-year medical students had been dissecting before the hurricane rotted in the heat. Rimma and her classmates would never dissect, missing out on a key ritual of becoming doctors.

Arriving at Kristy's house, Rimma opened the door to find that she had been lucky: Floodwater had risen just over the floor, soaking rugs, before draining out through the air ducts underneath. But a rancid odor filled the house. Rimma traced it to the kitchen—it was a pound of rotten butter, left on the counter from Kristy's popovers.

ST. VINCENT'S HOUSE was already up and serving people on the day that Rimma snuck back onto the island. Mr. Jackson had returned to Galveston two days after the storm as a first responder,

and he led St. Vincent's workers in making the House a hub for critical services. The Red Cross would drop off food, ice, and essential
supplies, and Mr. Jackson and his team would hand these supplies out
on the street.

With the medical students dispersed across the state and the future
of UTMB in question, the student-run free clinic would take weeks
to resume services. When it did, Kristy and the other student directors fanned out across the island trying to find their patients. They
knocked on doors, left flyers, and asked anybody who was around if
so-and-so patient had been seen. The houses they went to, mostly
north-side houses where the uninsured patients lived, were devastated. Most folks were gone, but some people were living in these
damaged, mold-infested places.

"I'm not sure how many people we actually found at home," Kristy
said, "but it was the minority." At one house, a man had ascites—
fluid in his belly, as Mr. Rose had had—so badly that Kristy could
diagnose it from the street. She encouraged him to come to St. Vincent's to see a doctor. "I'm not sure if he ever did," she said.

On the day the student-run free clinic opened again, a line of
patients was waiting out front at St. Vincent's House. Most of them
were longtime patients of Dr. Beach, the faculty sponsor for the
clinic. He had cared for some St. Vincent's patients for decades; they
had his cell phone number, and he had been able to let them know
about the clinic opening. Dr. Beach was the first volunteer to arrive
that day. When his patients saw him, they stood up and cheered.

MY INTERVIEW AT UTMB was rescheduled. It was finally held on
the campus of a medical school in Houston, about six weeks after the
storm. My friends in Galveston told me that things were still chaotic
on the island. There were still wrecked boats blocking some of the
minor roads, and many medical students had been sent to other hospitals across the state. The UTMB ER would not be up and running
until the following summer.

To orient us to Galveston at my off-island interview, the doctors showed a video that UTMB medical students had made. The video toured the hospital, the research buildings, and a bit of the island—all shot before the storm. Near the end of the video, a medical student popped out from behind a huge oak tree and said, "Galveston is verdant!" At that, the tall doctor in a suit and cowboy boots sitting next to me winced. Hundreds of oak trees on Galveston had been killed by the salty floodwaters.

I did not know at that time how much the hurricane and its aftermath would change my medical education. I did not know that the disaster, like Hurricane Katrina, would disproportionately affect the lives of poor people. Even if I had known that, I might have wondered what that could possibly have to do with me. The message the doctors gave us was that the hospital would surely be up and running in full service by the time my class started clinical rotations in our third year of medical school. If the hospital was running, it seemed, everything would be fine.

And anyway, Galveston was resilient. The town survived the Great Storm of 1900, and people there endured the years of recovery and rebuilding. The hospital had a century of history of taking care of those most in need. Surely, in this time of great need, UTMB and the city would rise to the occasion together.

My letter of acceptance to the MD/PhD program at Galveston arrived in the mail. When I opened it, I remembered watching the video footage of Hurricane Ike in the days after the storm. Reporters filmed the flooded north-side neighborhoods from a helicopter. In the middle of all that water, gas lines inside one of the houses had caught fire. The helicopter kept circling and circling around that lone house as it burned.

CHAPTER 5

THE FIRST THING SUSAN MCCAMMON AND HER HUSBAND replaced after the hurricane was their piano. Susan had been a musician long before she was a head-and-neck cancer surgeon, and by that point in her life she would tell you that the two practices—piano and surgery—were bound in her cerebellum, her muscles, her median nerve. You practice a particular movement over and over and then the thousandth time you do it, something changes—the notes become music, the surgery becomes a thing of beauty.

At UTMB, Susan had been a busy surgeon before the hurricane. She often ran two operating rooms at once. She trained junior surgeons, and she worked on a committee that tracked the funding for indigent patients. The goals of this committee seemed fairly clear: to provide as much care as possible to uninsured and indigent patients, using a limited pool of money. She also took classes at the Institute for the Medical Humanities, and derived satisfaction from being part of a hospital where her patients—because head-and-neck cancer patients are often working class or poor—got the same excellent care as insured patients. Busy as she was, Susan thrived. She felt herself at home in the total identity that medicine offered. Becoming a doctor was, for her, becoming a complete human being.

The early days after the storm were busy. Susan's first concern was to find her patients who were undergoing radiation. Head-and-neck cancer care is almost always multilevel: it can require chemotherapy, surgery, and radiation. Susan knew that any interruption in a radiation regimen—even just for a few days—could reduce her patients' chance of survival. A break in radiation therapy allows the stronger, radiation-resistant cancer cells to proliferate. So, along with her nurse, Susan immediately set about trying to catch up with these patients.

This was not easy. The island was still under evacuation orders, and Susan was in an extended-stay hotel in Dallas. Galveston-based patients were scattered all over the state and beyond. Landlines were not working and cell phone service was spotty; many of Susan's poorest patients—the ones who had lived on the streets or in the Salvation Army shelter on Galveston—didn't have cell phones. But she did what she could, and the MD Anderson Cancer Center in Houston agreed for a few weeks to accept UTMB cancer patients who were undergoing active radiation treatment at the time of the storm. So some found care there, some were treated elsewhere, and some patients could not be found.

Her next step was to find placements for her resident surgeons, so they could continue their training. Susan bought a fax machine and set up a temporary office in the hotel. She began calling residency programs around the state and beyond, asking them to take on the trainee surgeons from UTMB—at least for a month or two. This was all concrete work, and for a time, it kept Susan's mind off of the disaster.

Then she returned to the island, and to the clinic. Her house was wrecked. She still had her job. She had her car. She had her husband and her dog, which snored and drooled amid disaster, as he had always done before. The three of them moved into a second-story apartment near UTMB and hunkered down.

UTMB was also a mess, but miraculously, it stayed open. With John Sealy Hospital flooded, the administration began making arrangements for UTMB patients to be seen at mainland hospitals.

Susan and her colleagues were able to use clinic rooms and even operating rooms on the mainland, so many UTMB patients were able to continue getting the care they needed.

Susan felt lucky, even a little guilty, to have her job. In the weeks after the storm, nearly three thousand UTMB employees were abruptly fired under the reduction in force (RIF). In general, a state employee cannot be fired without reason and a type of due process. But in a crisis situation, the state is able to enact the RIF and fire people without other cause. Nobody on the ground could figure out the logic of the RIF—everyone from entry-level medical assistants to surgeons with thirty years of experience got RIFfed. As the waves of firings rolled out across the community, employees like Susan who still had jobs began to consider themselves very lucky. In fact, there was little for many of the doctors to do. With the main hospital shut down and many patients cut, suddenly professionals used to working eighty-hour weeks had a glut of time. How lucky, to be paid to do nothing while three thousand employees had been fired and the rest of the Gulf Coast struggled.

This luck, eventually, would have a silencing effect: those who now considered themselves lucky to have jobs at all mostly kept quiet about the changes at UTMB.

What Susan did not know, at that time, was how deeply those changes were affecting her patients. In the wake of the hurricane, UTMB administration had decided that the university could no longer provide unfunded care. And so Susan's indigent cancer patients had received a letter, signed by then-chancellor Ben Raimer, that began:

Dear [Name]:

We regret to inform you that UTMB physician Susan McCammon will be discontinuing her professional relationship with you due to the devastation caused by Hurricane Ike to UTMB's medical facilities and equipment. For this reason, we will no longer be able to offer you medical care at the University of Texas Medical Branch.

SUSAN LEARNED ABOUT the form letters when her patients began showing up at the clinic to ask her about it. They could not believe that Susan, who had cared for some of them for years, would abandon them. And the first time Susan took a letter from the damp and shaking hand of her patient, she could not believe it either. *Susan McCammon will be discontinuing her professional relationship with you . . .* The university couldn't do this, could they? Not to cancer patients. Not to people who surely would die without care.

In medical school, we learn that nonabandonment is essential to the practice of medicine. Once a doctor has established care with a patient, she cannot abruptly discontinue care without going through a process: explaining things to the patient, transferring their care to another doctor, continuing to provide care until the transfer is established. When patients get dire diagnoses, we learn to tell them that we will be beside them through the whole process. No matter how bad the disease, and no matter how brutal the treatment, we will not abandon them. This may be cold comfort to someone with an awful diagnosis, but the promise of nonabandonment is sometimes the only comfort we can give.

The notion that the university could compel a doctor to abandon her patients was shocking, and at first, Susan didn't believe it. She began making calls and asking questions, moving higher and higher up the chain of command. At every level, the answer seemed to be yes, they can do this. The state had cut funding for indigent care to UTMB, and in fact, the university had been gradually reducing funding for indigent care even in the years before Ike. Merle Lenihan, an ob-gyn doctor who formerly led the women's clinic at St. Vincent's House, worked with a community group called the Galveston County Free Care Monitoring Project to compile data showing that UTMB had been turning away more and more unfunded patients since 2005. Sixty-two percent of unfunded patients referred to UTMB had been accepted for care in 2007, the year before the storm.

By 2012, four years after Ike, only 9 percent were accepted. The total revenue dedicated to unfunded patients had steadily dropped, from 18 percent in 2005, down to 12.5 percent in 2007, and in 2009—a year after the storm—only 2.6 percent of UTMB revenue went to care for the uninsured.

These numbers, Merle argues, are out of step with UTMB's status as a public hospital. Nationwide, public hospitals—which not only are not-for-profit but also receive significant funding from state and federal governments—spent about 13 percent of revenue on unfunded care in 2012, on average. Merle's data suggests that the UTMB numbers were much more in line with averages in for-profit hospitals.*

Because charity care was already being cut before the storm, some felt that the hurricane provided the perfect screen for the university to fully enact a plan it had already begun. Others were more sympathetic to the university: It had undergone a costly evacuation for Hurricane Rita in 2005, withstood state budget cuts, and then been badly flooded during Ike. It was a miracle that UTMB was still running at all.

But politics aside, Susan could not fathom the logic of the form letter. It used her name. Because of that, her patients thought that she had chosen to abandon them. "Why won't you see me anymore?" they would ask—patients Susan loved. People whose bodies she had opened with her scalpel, and people with growing cancers who desperately needed the surgery she could offer. She would try to explain that it wasn't her, it wasn't her choice at all. But on some level it didn't matter: They were angry, and she was the person put before them. Her name was on the letter.

The second issue with the form letter was how neatly it blamed the abandonment of the poor patients on "the devastation caused by Hurricane Ike." On the mainland clinics, Susan noted the orderly

---

* These numbers come from the Galveston County Free Care Monitoring Project's independent review of UTMB financial reports. They are available online as "2012 Update: Achieving Reasonable Public Disclosure of Available Free and Reduced Cost Health Care in Galveston County, Texas," accessed May 17, 2016, http://gulfcoastinterfaith.org/yahoo_site_admin/assets/docs/2012_Update_Clearing_the_Fog.185150259.pdf.

procession of UTMB's paying patients in and out of operating rooms. The devastation caused by Hurricane Ike had not prevented UTMB from offering care to them.

The UTMB providers who spoke up about their charity patients were likely to be reminded of the RIF, and told that the cuts to charity care helped ensure that the institution could keep paying employees while the hospital recovered. And so the checks that came in felt not only unearned but also tainted, as if they came at the cost of patients' lives. Even so, UTMB providers managed to push the institution to fund one last visit with patients who would no longer be seen. In those final visits, Susan would do everything she could for her patients. She would tend to their wounds and their tumors as far as she could in her office. She would clean their tracheostomies—the tubes that went into some of their necks to help them breathe around a tumor—and write prescriptions for medications to control their pain. Her nurse would call around to area hospitals, trying to find a placement. But the limiting factors were chemotherapy, surgery, and radiation. Her patients needed these things to survive, and she could no longer offer them.

Who is a surgeon without her operating room? What does a good doctor do, when the institution she works for compels her to abandon patients who obviously need her help?

SUSAN BEGAN TO FIND her own answers to these questions by driving up the coast. Her Galveston patients were scattered, but many lived farther up the coast in areas that had not been flooded by Ike. These patients, too, had gotten the form letter. Susan often couldn't reach them by telephone, so in the weeks after Hurricane Ike, she began to climb into her little Volkswagen and drive out to find them. She was unaccustomed to all the free time Ike had granted her, and she began to fill it with the practice of medicine.

The weather was beautiful then—sunny and cool, the most perfect October you could dream of after your town was destroyed.

It felt almost like a vacation for a while, leaving the wreckage of Galveston behind and driving through the seaside towns, listening to Bach's Goldberg Variations or his Sonatas for Viola da Gamba and Harpsichord. These towns were startlingly intact compared with Galveston. The oak trees were alive, the restaurants were open, people had lawn chairs and swing sets in their yards. Susan would drive to the nearest point she could find listed as her patient's address. If she couldn't find the house, she would start asking around at corner stores and churches, until someone knew where her patient lived. Susan's patients spanned the width of American poverty: some were in houses, and some were in trailers, and some were in garage apartments with dirt floors, where the electricity came from an extension cord and running water could be an issue. They welcomed her in, and she began to learn that every little house, no matter how humble, can feel just like home. Susan would duck through the low door of a trailer, and someone would offer her a cup of tap water. The sick bed often took up most of the space inside, and so afterward she would be invited to sit in the folding chairs out front. She was conscious of her own comparative wealth, and grateful for her modest car that was not too shabby to seem doctorly, but still wouldn't stick out in any neighborhood.

Oddly, Susan's patients did not seem surprised to see her. It was as if they had been sitting at the edge of the bed, waiting for her to walk in. There were people at every stage of treatment: people who had just been diagnosed, to whom, weeks before, Susan had explained that they had a great chance of surviving. There were people who were bedridden, with feeding tubes in their stomachs and tracheostomies in their throats. And there were those in between—some who had gotten surgery already, and some who had not. "So what are we going to do, doc?" they would ask her. "What's our plan?"

That is when the easy autumn feeling grew thin and shaky, because the truth is that Susan did not know exactly what to do. Some of her patients were convinced that the interruption in care was a temporary thing, and that UTMB would take them back as soon as it could.

Others had already begun to seek care elsewhere. Still others were too sick to do anything at all. She had to tell them that it was true: she would no longer be able to treat their cancer.

Susan's patients would ask her what would happen to them if they didn't get care, and this was even worse. Head-and-neck cancer is often inexorable. If untreated, it chokes you to death, or it grows back into your brain, or it erodes into a major artery so you suddenly bleed to death. You can hemorrhage out of your mouth and nose and drown in your own blood unless there is a doctor right at hand to put in a tube that will block the blood from flowing down into the lungs. Susan began forcing herself to tell the truth—not all those details, but the truth. "You'll die," she would say. "You'll die because of this. I know I said you had a 70 percent chance of being alive five years from now, but that was with treatment. Without treatment, your mortality rate within a year will be 100 percent."

This is not an easy thing to say, and sometimes she failed. She would dance around the issue, talking about county indigent care plans and applications to Medicaid, even when she knew those plans weren't going to work. The conversations were sometimes circuitous. So then she tried to force herself to say it very strongly—"You will die"—and that was awful also. It was too much. Sometimes the conversations were arduous, two-hour-long affairs, with the patients saying, "Tell me again how it is that I'm not going to get care." And so she would try to repeat it. A time or two, she arrived at a patient's house and sat silently in her car for a few minutes, then turned around and drove back to Galveston, too heartsick to have the conversation again.

Still, she felt that these conversations had to happen face-to-face. She could not fathom the form letter, the innocuous language that in fact meant bleeding, suffocation, death. Her patients deserved at the very least to hear it in person, to have it made plain. So she returned to their homes and to these impossible conversations.

Susan was in unfamiliar territory, beyond the guidelines of how physicians discuss death. As a surgeon, she had been trained to confront bad diagnoses. She knew how to tell a patient that treatment was not working, and how to tell a patient that her disease could not be cured. Many of her patients had died before, because cancer patients often do. But this felt different; she could not blame the cancer itself, the disease that humbles all of medicine. The situation felt unnatural and she wasn't sure who to blame. The insurance system? The state? The hurricane? As an employee on the UTMB payroll, Susan felt implicated in the withdrawal of care, and so at times she blamed herself. She felt like a useless novelty: a surgeon who could not operate, a cancer doctor who could not cure.

She had some idea, however, that she could stand by her patients. She could go to their houses, and lay on her hands, and comfort them. She could clean their wounds, change their tubes, write prescriptions for their pain. Each encounter began with the washing of hands, and sometimes to wash her hands Susan had to begin by washing the dishes in the sink and then putting them away, because her patients were alone and sick and things like dishes had been forgotten. So she would do that, the dishes and her hands, and then begin. As strange as this was, it was also deeply familiar, the same old rituals of doctoring acted out in a trailer park outside Beaumont: clean hands, vital signs, history taking, care. Sometimes a neighbor or a neighbor's kid would be sick, and Susan would see them, too.

Yet some of her patients did not want this. They did not want her comfort, or the laying on of hands, or a doctor who follows the ethical imperative of patient nonabandonment. They wanted surgery, radiation, chemotherapy, and cure. They wanted to live.

Susan understood. Maybe there was even relief when they got angry, because partly she wanted to be punished for her sins: her job, her health, her full paycheck at a time when so few patients were getting operations that she could drive up the coast on her days off. She wondered if the whole thing—the laying on of hands, the comfort, the nonabandonment—was just a complicated way of soothing her own guilt.

And so she tried to fix things, to work within the system. But understanding the system was like grasping at smoke. You would see for a moment a way to answer the questions—*Why are my patients dying? What do we do?*—and then it would disappear. There had been a time, before the storm, when Susan's work on the committee that followed charity care in the hospital had felt clear and right: obviously, there were limited funds, but the goal was to get as much care as possible to as many patients as they could.

After the storm it was not like that. Everything became contingent, and every plan unraveled. The committee didn't meet for a month. Then the membership changed, and finally after a long time of Susan asking questions that nobody could or would answer, the committee was dissolved. When it was reformed, Susan was not on it. And by that time she was too heartbroken to fight it. She did not believe that UTMB was trying to offer care to the indigent.* She was exhausted.

Most of Susan's friends and mentors counseled her to step away. The situation, they said, was untenable. Some told her to focus instead on public health—preventing cancer by preventing smoking—or laboratory research, or policy change. They said she would burn out. They said that a surgeon's duty ends when she can no longer do surgery. They said she should leave. There were plenty of opportunities to leave, as other academic medical centers were actively recruiting UTMB doctors. Many good people left UTMB, but Susan couldn't. She kept returning to the particular, those particular people in whose bodies the policy and public health and personal story seemed to crystalize, and who were dying in makeshift houses up and down the Texas coast.

The whole experience has not made her a better person, she thinks. Rather, it has made her feel heavier, weighed down by the constant presence of suffering that she cannot ameliorate, and which comes from sources that feel artificial. As complicated and mysterious as cancer is, she understands the place it holds in life. Cancer is tangible,

---

* In 2014, UTMB president David Callender finally stated publicly that charity was no longer part of UTMB's "core mission."

vicious, and real; bureaucracy is otherwise. It is deliberately designed to obfuscate, to be the smoke in the air that nobody can grasp.

IT WAS JANUARY when Susan's patients began to die.

There is a dividing line in head-and-neck cancer, between people who have tracheostomies and people who don't. The trach patients have a protected airway, a tube that goes from their throat down to their lungs. But the patients without trachs do not, so when the cancer closes up their throat, they begin to starve and suffocate. They move more and more slowly, breathe less and less. Then one day they get laryngitis or a cold, and their airway collapses suddenly, and they die, as did several of Susan's patients. Their families would say they had died in their sleep, and it was a result of airway collapse.

The sound that breath makes when a patient's airway is collapsing is called "stridor"—a harsh, wheezing sound. If these patients could have gotten to an ER with an on-call surgeon in that critical moment when they had stridor, they would have been given an emergency tracheostomy. But for a time, the ER in Galveston was closed and Beaumont or Houston hospitals were far away—a life-flight away. In rural Texas, as Susan would point out, the barriers to care often begin well before the hospital.

Patients with trachs died in other ways. Their cancer metastasized to their livers or lungs, or extended directly back into their skulls and killed them. One patient's tumor eroded into his carotid artery, and he bled out massively into his own body and died. Others died of what Susan calls the "cancer dwindles"—they grew thinner and thinner as the cancer demanded more and more of the energy that their body could produce, and finally they were bedridden and then they died. In an awful way, it was educational for Susan to see all this, what we refer to as the "natural history" of the disease that she had been trained to cure.

Susan did not attend their funerals. She never has been one for patient funerals, in part because she feels that as the doctor she draws too much attention at them. Family members come up to thank her, when they should be able to simply be immersed in their own grief.

She also feels that her patients cross some kind of bright line in dying, between being under her care and being under the care of their families, or God. She is not religious. But she sees all her patients who have died very clearly; she imagines them all side by side in a high pew in the Government Street Presbyterian Church in Mobile, Alabama, looking down. The upholstery there is gold and velvety, and the light makes golden dust motes. Susan's patients are looking down and she can see their faces, and they have something to teach her. Though in these cases, as often, she is not yet sure what the lesson is.

CHAPTER 6

THE SUMMER AFTER THAT JANUARY WHEN SUSAN'S PATIENTS began to die, I moved to Galveston. I spent the summer taking PhD courses at the Institute for the Medical Humanities and waiting for August, when medical school would begin. All summer, I heard stories about St. Vincent's. Margaret was a student director there. She and her friends told St. Vincent's stories at the cookouts and potlucks that populate the summertimes of medical school. I heard about a patient dying from cancer of the liver who couldn't get on the transplant list—presumably because he had once used heroin. But could it actually be because he was uninsured? And a woman diagnosed with schizophrenia who refused all medications and kept getting arrested for hollering in the street. And a medical student who was trying to treat a circle of men who kept reinfecting one another with syphilis. "I need to just get all ten of them into clinic at once," he joked, "so we can make sure they're all treated simultaneously."

Who were these schizophrenic, syphilitic, cancerous uninsured heroin-injecting criminals in my backyard? They sounded like strangers to me.

One Thursday afternoon, about a month before I was set to start medical school classes, Margaret loaned me a white coat and took me to the clinic. We drove across the north side of the island, away from

UTMB and past downtown to where St. Vincent's House stands among a swath of devastated blocks and empty lots. Amid the blankness of the north side after Ike, the House was buzzing with activity. Cars lined the street out front, and more people were walking or riding beat-up bicycles toward the clinic. I could hear music playing on the outdoor speakers. Unlike anything around it, the House had shrubbery: green bushes planted along the outside wall. In the years to come, St. Vincent's would get even brighter: murals would spread from the main building to the basketball court to the sidewalk out front. A Hope Mile with exercise equipment would be dedicated for walking, and a community garden would spring up on the grounds.

Margaret shepherded me up the outdoor stairs to the second story of the House. We opened the door and stepped right into the clinic waiting room, where a dozen people glanced up to see us enter. There they were: the uninsured.

The uninsured were reading magazines, glancing down at phones, or talking with relatives who had come along to pass the minutes (or hours) of waiting to see a doctor. A little girl slept with her head in her mother's lap, and one couple nervously held hands. They looked ordinary to me because they were: At that time in Texas, 26 percent of all people were uninsured—including many folks I knew from Port Aransas. Including my brother Matt, who had grown up to be a commercial fisherman.

So my first impression of St. Vincent's patients was one of ordinariness. The cancerous schizophrenic criminals in the waiting room of my imagination turned out to just be ordinary people. If I feared anything from these people, it was that they would see through me. They would notice that my white coat was too big, and realize I knew little about medicine.

It struck me over the years that St. Vincent's House, when the student clinic is in full swing, is divided. If you walk into the waiting room and turn left, into the offices of the House, you will find that most of the people who work and volunteer there are African American. If you walk into the waiting room and turn right, down the hall into the clinic, most of the medical students and doctors are white. The waiting room, where the patients aggregate, is mixed. Historically, St. Vincent's House had been a place where black workers and volunteers served a largely black clientele. The clinic was a bit of an anomaly—Dr. Beach, the volunteer doctor who oversaw it, was white. And the student volunteers were a diverse group, but were (like me) still mostly white. According to Mr. Jackson, this was a cause of some concern at the House. Community members aware of the history of medical and scientific experimentation on American blacks worried that the medical students were "experimenting" on the patients. And in a way this was true. We weren't doing scientific research there, but we were learning.

After Ike, the demographics of Galveston Island changed dramatically. The historically black neighborhoods on Galveston took the brunt of the flooding, and many black residents were forced off the island. Galveston's political leaders fought against rebuilding the public housing that had been vital to many of the people of St. Vincent's. The House began to serve more white people. This transition bothered some of the African American workers and volunteers at St. Vincent's. "When stuff started to change, folks said, 'Gosh, we serving the enemy. They wouldn't serve us, now we serving them,'" Mr. Jackson told me.

But the people of the House did not stop serving Galveston. "Folks come here for hope, and whatever we materially can provide for them, that's our job," Mr. Jackson said. "That's what we do."

In my first months at St. Vincent's, I never turned left. I hurried through the waiting room toward the safety of the clinical area, where students in short white coats huddled around charts like birds around a handful of seed. That was where, in the clinical space, I belonged.

THE FIRST PATIENT I SAW that first day at St. Vincent's had a most ordinary problem: she needed a preemployment physical exam.

I trailed after a third-year medical student who called the patient back
into an exam room and began to rattle off questions from memory.
Had she had fevers? Chills? Sweating? Dizziness? Cough? Coughing
any blood? Pain in her belly? Tingling in her arms and legs? Waking
up at night to pee? Did she feel short of breath when she lay down?
How many pillows did she sleep on? The questions went on and on.
She was a healthy twenty-six-year-old. I was amazed that this student
knew all those questions from memory. I would learn them soon
as the review of systems: a handy tool that screens for symptoms in
all the organ systems of the body. I sat silently on a chair beside the
other student and let the questions wash past me, just as the tour of
the clinic—explaining everything from which antibiotics we had to
how to check blood sugar to where the speculums are stored—would
wash over me. The student talked a mile a minute, and I knew I
would never remember it all. I didn't even know exactly what blood
sugar was.

After a quick physical exam and a check-in with the doctor, we
signed that first patient's note and sent her on her way.

"She wasn't your usual St. Vincent's patient," the student told me
as she disappeared back out toward the waiting room. "Most of the
people you see here will be really sick."

AT THE END OF AUGUST, I got my own white coat in a massive
ceremony with my class of 230 new medical students. As the first
class of medical students to join UTMB after Hurricane Ike, we were
told that we were a symbol of hope for the whole island. We got little
gold pins for our white coats that read, "UTMB: We Stop for No
Storm." My parents drove down to Galveston for the ceremony, and
barbecued a celebratory brisket in the yard of the yellow house.

Along with our white coats and our hurricane pins, each new medical student received an identical black backpack with the UTMB
logo. We all used these backpacks, and we all had the same class
schedule. So when classes began, we would travel in a pack from lec-

ture hall to anatomy lab and back across campus to a building called Graves, which had rooms for labs and small-group discussion classes called PBL: problem-based learning.

The cases we discussed were based on actual patients who'd been seen at UTMB. In my first PBL class, we discussed a patient who required plastic surgery to repair a wound he'd received while fleeing from the police.

"Okay, so what's the anatomy you need to know for this surgery?" our group leader asked the ten of us gathered in the discussion room. We could hear the hum and thud of construction on the first story below us, which had flooded during Ike.

"He's in prison, right?" one of my classmates asked. She was a white woman from outside Dallas who had worked in an emergency room before medical school. She knew the definitions of all the medical words, and snapped out answers before the rest of us had time to think. "I don't think we need to know any anatomy at all," she said.

"What?" I said.

"I mean, he broke the law," she said. "Why should he get medical care?"

I expected the class to erupt in protest, but there was a general shrug. Finally I said, "Well, the Constitution prevents cruel and unusual punishment. So that's why prisoners get medical care."

"Maybe so, but I don't have to treat them," she said.

At first, all my classmates seemed like her: young, anxious, and conservative. There were women who woke up at seven a.m. and meticulously curled their eyelashes before a long morning of dissecting a human cadaver. There were men who lived in an all-male medical fraternity known for cheating on tests. There was an annual "white trash"–themed party. (*What am I supposed to do, go as myself?*) These students seemed poised to become the kind of doctors that Frank and I had imagined, and I felt like the only outsider.

I could not imagine that woman from Dallas with all the right answers working to help a patient at the prison hospital on the UTMB campus. She would, though; we all would. In the beginning I stood apart, watching the sea of classmates in identical backpacks flowing from class to class. There on campus, medical school did not feel revelatory, life altering, or transcendent. It felt like junior high.

I GRAVITATED TOWARD ST. VINCENT'S, where Margaret and her cool friends were running the show. As soon as I learned a new skill on campus—part of the physical exam, or history taking—I could put it into practice as a volunteer at the clinic. I started out shadowing the more advanced students, then seeing patients along with an upper-level student, and then along with a fellow first-year.

One of the first patients I interviewed was a young man from El Salvador who had a rash on the backs of his hands. We spoke Spanish. My conversational Spanish was good, and in a class for bilingual medical students, I had learned how to do the review of systems in Spanish. "Have you had any palpitations—when you noticed your heart beating in your chest?" I asked. I happily rattled off the questions about coughing blood, trouble with urinating, and difficulty maintaining erections. I was so proud to know these terms in Spanish that I didn't feel embarrassed at all.

The only trouble I discovered in the review of systems was tinnitus: ringing in his ears.

"Okay, when did that start?" I asked him brightly.

"When I was fourteen," he said.

"And what was going on then?" I asked. "Were you listening to a lot of loud music?"

"Not really," he said. "I was in the war."

"The war," I repeated.

"I guess it was because there was a lot of shooting, and my gun was very close to my ear."

He had come from El Salvador, where a bloody civil war that I knew little about had raged for thirteen years. He had been forced to join a paramilitary group after his father was disappeared and his sisters were murdered. And now he was in Galveston, working for a landscaping company.

After the review of systems, I moved to the physical exam. The rash on the backs of his hands was red and a little bit flaky. I wondered if it could be related to his work, but wasn't sure. I needed to ask the doctor.

His heart sounded good, and his lungs sounded fine. On his right calf, there was a huge scar. "Where did you get this scar?" I asked.

"In El Salvador," he said.

"What happened?"

"Well, one day they were shooting at me, and I fell down a mountain."

If I hadn't been a first-year student then, I probably would not have asked all the questions in the review of systems. I would have done a focused physical exam instead of a full physical, and not looked much further than the rash on his hands. I might not have heard his story about being forced to become a soldier when he was still a child.

Is this important, though? None of that information changed how we cared for his rash: a simple steroid cream and a recommendation to wear gloves at work. It was the most ordinary of problems, and the cure was easy.

As I was leaving the room, he reminded me of the tinnitus. "Do you have medicine for this ringing in my ears?" he asked.

I didn't.

"It's okay," he said, shrugging his shoulders with his palms toward the ceiling. "It's really nothing."

OUTSIDE OF CLINIC, I spent most of my time either dissecting a cadaver or frantically memorizing the names and locations of nerves, arteries, and muscles. I had hoped to be disturbed by anatomy lab. If it really upset me to dissect a dead person, then surely I was normal: human, healthy, and emotionally intact. But instead of being disturbed, I was fascinated. Anatomy lab itself rapidly became normal: normal to cut flesh and saw bone, normal to hold a human heart in my hands, normal to slide my own gloved hand under the skin of a dead woman's arm.

There is a history to anatomy lab. The earliest anatomy texts we know of were written by Egyptian physicians around 2000 BC. Physicians have been dissecting ever since—even though human dissection has been, in many societies, illegal. The most famous dissector of them all was Andreas Vesalius, a brilliant and progressive anatomist who lived in the 1500s. Before Vesalius, both Ottoman and European physicians had trusted the work of Galen, a Greek physician who died around the year 200. Galen's anatomy text was thought infallible, and physicians from around Vesalius's time let technicians dissect while they themselves stood high above the body, reading from Galen's text. It was not fit for a physician to dirty his hands in a human body—not when real knowledge came on high from the Greeks.

The young Vesalius showed doctors another path to knowledge. In his early twenties, he set about making meticulous dissections that proved that Galen had misidentified several structures. In some cases—as in Galen's claim that tiny pores in the heart allowed the blood to circulate from left to right—Vesalius found that Galen was completely wrong. This was a significant challenge to the physicians of the sixteenth century. Vesalius's work called on physicians to descend, and to look for truth within the body itself.

As Vesalius grew famous, he dissected before audiences—both medical professionals and the curious public. Many of the bodies that he used to make his great discoveries were those of condemned, and recently executed, criminals.

Why did Vesalius dissect criminals? In some cases, to be dissected by physicians after death was part of the punishment for a crime. To dissect a body is to desecrate it—literally, to take away its sacredness.

In my experience, dissection was indeed desecration: If we students felt a holy awe and terror on the first day we approached the cadavers we would dissect, that awe faded as the bodies were sliced, chopped, and disarticulated. We approached a body that had a kind of sacredness, and we dissected it into its very material parts.

Western doctors would shy away from dissecting people we know and love, because they are so sacred to us. Strangers are less sacred. And those who seem to have committed some great sin against society fall into the group most vulnerable to dissection: those whose lives seem, to others, to have no sacredness. And because the lives of condemned criminals were not considered sacred, it hardly mattered what befell their cadavers.

Yet the knowledge gained from their bodies was meant to enrich us all. In the introduction to his famous *On the Fabric of the Human Body*, Vesalius writes to Emperor Charles V, whose patronage he needed in order to get his book published. "Nothing could be produced more pleasing or welcome to your majesty," Vesalius writes, "than research in which we recognize the body and the spirit, as well as a certain divinity that issues from a harmony of the two, and finally in our own selves." Knowledge gained from the disarticulation of criminals could shed light on the spiritual body of an emperor.

If my time in the anatomy lab was spiritual—showing me the divinity in the union of body and spirit—this spirituality came only in flashes. I was fascinated by anatomy, but mostly unmoved. Without the breath of life, the body before me had become a useful object.

Just as dissection has a history, the dissected bodies have a politics. In the early years of the United States, cadavers for dissection in medical schools came almost exclusively from communities of color.* Doctors in the Southwest dissected the bodies of Native Americans. Slave owners sold the bodies of enslaved people, who were considered property even after death, to medical schools. African American soldiers who died in the Civil War were dissected by Army surgeons eager to hone their craft. Because the white medical profession did

* Edward C. Halperin, "The Poor, the Black, and the Marginalized as the Source of Cadavers in United States Anatomical Education," *Clinical Anatomy* 20 (2007): 489–495.

not recognize the sacredness—the symbolic life—of people of color, their bodies were seen as fit for dissection.*

In some cases, enslaved people were actually made to dig up and steal the bodies of other African Americans. In 1852, the Medical College of Georgia bought an enslaved man named Grandison Harris. Harris was put to the task of snatching the bodies of other black people from the local cemetery. Through his work in the medical school, Harris grew knowledgeable about dissection. After emancipation, he became a teacher at the very medical college where he had been enslaved.

It is now—as it was then—illegal to steal bodies for dissection. It is also technically illegal to sell bodies and body parts. So, in American medical schools today, cadavers are donated. Some are donated by people who are grateful for the medical care they received, and want to give something back to the profession and to other patients. Some are donated by people who don't want to—or can't—burden their families with the expense of cremation or burial. Websites seeking people to donate their bodies to science often emphasize that all costs will be covered. ("MedCure arranges services at NO COST including: transportation, cremation, and return of cremated remains to family in approximately 6 to 12 weeks or a scattering at sea," one such website reads.)

There is no hard data on what percentage of donated bodies come from people living in poverty. Nor is there hard data on race. In fact, the ongoing issue of medical abuses of African Americans dissuades some people in the black community from donating. A 2004 survey of Maryland households found that people who agreed with the statement "White patients receive better care in hospitals than other racial or ethnic groups" were much less likely to consider donation.† Yet the economic incentive for donation means

---

* Jason E. Glenn, "Dehumanization, the Symbolic Gaze, and the Production of Biomedical Knowledge," in *Black Knowledges/Black Struggles: Essays in Critical Epistemology*, ed. Jason R. Ambroise and Sabine Broeck (Liverpool, UK: Liverpool University Press, 2015), 112–144.

† Boulware et al., "Whole-Body Donation for Medical Science: A Population-Based Survey," *Clinical Anatomy* 17, no. 7 (October 2004): 570–577.

that some people who do donate are impelled by poverty as much as, or rather than, gratitude.

Medical students are taught to think of the grateful donors—the ones who wanted to give something back to the medical profession. We are encouraged to consider their cadavers as a "gift."

There is a tyranny in giving, though—especially the gift that cannot be equaled. "How can I ever repay this gift?" I asked my friend Katie. We were sitting on the front porch of the yellow house one evening after her day in the hospital, and mine in the anatomy lab.

"You can't," she said. "It's impossible. It's too great. You just have to learn as much as you can, and try to pay it back by becoming a really good doctor." In Katie's eyes, it was right that medical students should begin our learning under the debt of a gift we cannot repay.

I find Katie's point beautiful and right. But another side of this politics concerns those patients—those people, those bodies—who were too poor to pay for burial or cremation. Already in anatomy lab, we medical students begin by learning on the bodies of the poor. Knowledge gained from them makes us into doctors: I would never again look at a shoulder without being able to imagine the muscles, bones, nerves, and arteries that course under the skin. I learned to see as a doctor sees, from these particular bodies.

Were the people whose bodies I dissected victims of symbolic death while they were still living? Were they poor? I had no way of knowing. Along with my classmates, I disarticulated the body completely. Lungs and guts went into a sack. Skin was removed. The body was chopped in half at the pelvis. The top of the skull was sawed off and the brain was removed. (I did this. I move into the passive voice to describe it, but the truth is: I did it. I held the circulating saw as chips of bone flew into the air around me.) We sawed off an areola, sliced through an eyeball, cut penises in half to see the chambers of flesh inside. If these people had been poor, it did not matter to me, because all I saw was the body in its parts.

This is the precise strangeness of learning to see like a doctor. If you believe hard enough in the truths of biochemistry and anatomy, what surrounds them—people with their suffering, the politics of a society that lay this particular body into your hands—seems not to matter at all.

One week, the air-conditioning across UTMB, which had been tetchy since Ike, failed completely. Classes were canceled, and our anatomy professors spent those days dumping ice into the coffinlike steel tanks that held our cadavers. These tanks work with a winch on both ends: two medical students pull the winch on either end of the tank, and the cadaver rises from a bath of preserving fluid ("cadaver juice") to the top for the day's dissection. When we winched up our bodies after the air-conditioning was restored, the tanks were so full of melted ice that cadaver juice slushed out all over our shoes. In the chest of our cadaver, between the pectoral muscles and the space where the lungs had been removed, a fluffy white mold had blossomed in the heat. I wiped it away with a gloved hand, and we carried on with the dissection.

IF EVERY YEAR OF MY LIFE were like the first year of medical school, my tombstone would read, "She studied." Seeing the body in its parts seemed to obliterate the rest of the body's meaning, but studying hard enough to keep up in medical school seemed to obliterate the entire world. As I slipped out of contact with friends, my old life began to feel impossibly far away. Caitlin commented that I sounded "very professional" when I would leave a message on her voice mail. Whoever I had been before was gone, but I wasn't anything like a doctor yet. I was just a shade of a woman, struggling to memorize a thousand facts.

St. Vincent's was my relief. I would make it to the clinic once a week, or once every two weeks. At St. Vincent's, I could lose myself in blissful concentration on another person's problems.

As the older student had promised on my first day at the clinic, many of these problems were complicated. I saw a patient with heart failure who could not walk half a block without gasping for breath. I saw people with schizophrenia and bipolar disorder, and sat stunned as they described the changes in their thinking that the mental illness brought. I learned to carefully check the feet of every diabetic patient for the sores that they might not notice after their skin had become numb from the damage of the disease.

Many St. Vincent's patients were still suffering from the effects of Hurricane Ike, even though the storm was now a year behind us. One woman with an anxiety disorder told me that her panic attacks were more frequent since she'd been forced to move into a crowded house with her cousins. Another patient told my friend that her asthma was worse because there was a boat in her house. The boat had crashed through a wall during the flood, and she was still living in the moldy wreckage.

One Saturday afternoon, I cared for a homeless man who walked into the examination room with three plastic bags full of belongings. His name was Mr. Tran, and he had diabetes. I wanted to know if his medications were working, but what he really wanted to know was why I wasn't married.

"No ring?" he commented.

"No sir," I said. "Do you ever get tingling in your hands and feet?"

"Yes I do, in my toes," he said. "But you are so lovely."

"How long has that been going on?" I asked.

"A long time," he said. "You know, I am not married either."

"Okay. A long time—do you mean weeks, months, years?"

"Oh, for years," he answered. "I'm homeless, but I am very strong. I'm a gentleman." He smiled, leaning back against the wall of the exam room. It was a truly joyful smile.

"I'm sure you are, sir," I said. "I'm going to check your blood sugar now."

"Okay, well, think it over," he said.

"You're going to feel a little sting in this finger when the needle goes in," I said.

By that time, I had checked the blood sugar on a dozen patients, so I felt comfortable with the procedure. I cleaned his finger with an alcohol swab, and pressed a tiny needle into the fleshy part of the fingertip. With my gloved hand, I pressed a bead of blood out of the puncture, then scooped that bead into a special strip that inserts it into the handheld glucometer. The glucometer gives a number— blood sugars under 120 are normal for someone who hasn't eaten recently.

This time, the glucometer gave no number. It read, "Err." So I tried again. When it said "Err" again, I excused myself to check with Katie, who was directing the clinic that day. She told me to try again with a different glucometer, which also gave an error message. Having pricked this man's finger three times, we decided to draw blood for a hemoglobin A1c—a test that shows the average blood sugar level over the past three months—and leave it at that. We wouldn't change his medications based on a single blood sugar reading, anyway.

So Mr. Tran gathered his plastic bags and left, smiling at me joyfully and asking me once again to consider his proposal. "We'll see you back at clinic in three weeks," I said.

After I left the clinic that afternoon, Katie called me on my cell phone. "Did you get a phone number for Mr. Tran?" she asked me. I hadn't. I had assumed he didn't have a phone because he was homeless—not a good assumption.

"Did his lab results come in already?" I asked.

"No," she said. "It's that glucometer. I checked with Dr. Beach, and he says it probably read 'Error' because Mr. Tran's glucose was over 600." A glucose level that high is an emergency. If we had caught it, we would have sent Mr. Tran to the ER at UTMB. But we missed it. Our supervising doctor hadn't caught it because the glucose reading was an afterthought—something he'd reminded me to do after he had already seen the patient and signed his prescriptions.

Katie spent the afternoon calling anywhere she thought Mr. Tran might be—the Salvation Army shelter, the Our Daily Bread group that feeds the homeless, the Jesse Tree organization. Nobody knew where he was. Then she drove around the island looking for him, but she never found him.

When I imagined making mistakes in medicine, I always imagined something more dramatic—cutting through an artery in surgery, or making a wrong diagnosis. I didn't imagine these pedestrian mistakes, like forgetting to report the results of a urine sample or forgetting to get a phone number. Even more so, I didn't foresee that such mundane errors could cost my patients their lives. And, as it is with so many patients I have seen as a student, I don't know what happened with Mr. Tran. I hope he found help.

ANATOMY ENDED WITH A BRUTAL multiple-choice exam and a lab practical. The only way to describe our studying before this test is to say that it was constant.

For the practical, we gathered in the anatomy lab, tense and silent. We each received a number, and walked to the tank with that number on it. At each tank, a structure in the body had been tagged with a colored pin. We had to name the structure, or its function, or answer another question about it. We had roughly one minute per tank, and then a buzzer would ring, signaling us to rotate to the next tank.

I moved from tank to tank at the buzzer, scribbling down answers for my exam. At one, I answered the question quickly and confidently, so I had a moment to glance up around the lab.

All was silent. By this time, the bodies were utterly dissected. Here and there across the clean stainless-steel surfaces of the lab, a human leg was strung up with its muscles flayed. On one tank, a dissected hand sat alone, its rose-colored nail polish still perfect. Another had a woman's pelvis, split in half with a yellow pin stuck in the labia minora. Sawed-open heads stared out from sockets dissected down to show the tiny muscles that move the eye.

All of these were things that I could see, recognize, and name. And when I looked out over my classmates, I noticed that each of them was as haggard as I. We were pale from studying, with shadows under our eyes and shoulders slumped as we stared at the corpses before us. One woman's brow was furrowed and her eyes were closed as if in pain. I could name that, too: it was suffering.

The buzzer sounded, and we moved as one group to the next cadaver.

THE DAY AFTER THE FINAL, I went to St. Vincent's. I needed something good, something that made me feel like medicine was alive and human.

That something good came in the form of a fifty-five-year-old woman with high blood pressure. She worked in a hotel on the seawall, and shopped at the same grocery store I go to. She'd been sent to St. Vincent's after doctors at a community health fair had noticed that her blood pressure was high. And she had spent two weeks worrying while she waited for her appointment.

"My father had high blood pressure, and he died of a heart attack," she told me. "I'm terrified. I have kids myself. My son is at College of the Mainland, and I have a little grandbaby on the way."

I took her history and found that her blood pressure was still high. I didn't see any signs of advanced disease, though: her heart sounded fine, her feet and ankles were normal. Then I talked with the doctor, and listened as he slowly and calmly walked her through everything she needed to know: what high blood pressure means, what the risks are, what she could do to reduce her blood pressure on her own, and how we would help treat it.

"Good job coming in," he told her. "At this stage, we should be able to treat you and help prevent any heart problems." I walked out with the doctor, and returned to the exam room with her prescription in my hand.

"Here you go," I said.

"Where can I get it filled?" she asked.

"It should be four dollars at Walmart, so I'd go there," I said.

And at that, she burst into tears. "Thank you so much," she said.

She touched my skinny wrist where it stuck out from the rolled-back sleeve of my short white coat. "God bless you."

It was an ordinary problem, and the treatment was simple. I felt I had done so little. I knew so little—I wasn't even sure I had passed my anatomy exam. But when this woman stood and reached out to hug me, I opened my arms.

CHAPTER 7

Not all my learning happened at St. Vincent's, of course. In the Practice of Medicine (POM) course, I was formally taught to do what a doctor actually does: physical exams, history taking, writing notes. I learned how to counsel people about cigarette smoking, when to call Child Protective Services, and why one shouldn't have sex with her patients. (Answer: because it's in the Hippocratic oath.) POM is a two-year course that begins the first week of medical school and lasts until we start on the wards in third year.

At St. Vincent's, I had already learned a lot of the skills that were taught in POM. But POM was a protected space. There, I could do what a medical student really should: practice. Not on real patients. Not on poor people who were bewilderingly ill and had no other choice but to see a student. In POM, I could practice on well-paid actors from the Galveston community.

These actors are called "standardized patients" or "SPs," and they learn to act out illness by script. Like the students, they learn what is proper in the physical exam and in history taking. And so, after each encounter with a student, the standardized patients would grade us on our skills.

Many of these encounters took place in an elaborate theater: a wing of our lecture-hall building that was designed to look like a clinic. There were cameras in each room, so that our professors could watch us interact with patients and—I happen to know—make fun of us.

Some of my friends from the Institute for the Medical Humanities had side jobs working as standardized patients. They had to put my name on a list of friends so that I wouldn't ever walk into a fake clinic room and find them pretending to worry over a sick (fake) baby or trying to avoid disclosing a (fake) exposure to gonorrhea. But through them, I got the scoop on the SPs. Yes, they and our professors were laughing at us in the room with the video monitors. How could they not?

There was the student who had clearly been taught the "clinical pearl" that he must reach out to touch his patient if the patient is upset. He reached out and placed a comforting hand directly on one standardized patient's inner thigh. There was the student who told one standardized patient that her vaginal discharge was "awesome, because we can totally treat that." There were plenty who turned bright red at any mention of a vagina.

As second-year POM students, we saw not only SPs playing straightforward cases, but also what were euphemistically called "complicated cases." Lots of the complicated cases had to do with sex, because medical students are a virginal bunch—at least in Texas. We're great at studying. Really great! Not always so great at the rest of life. In the 1970s, they used to show pornography to medical students so they would have some idea of what was going on when patients described their sexual activity.

Other cases were just socially complicated. There was the patient addicted to pain medication, the delusional young mother who was deliberately making her child sick, and the pair of Uruguayan American brothers who tried desperately to convince me not to reveal to their imaginary father that he had pancreatic cancer. The brothers were wonderful. They screamed and shook their hands in the air, and one of them—for reasons I will never understand—had fake blood all over his forehead. (I assume it was fake.)

"In Uruguay," he shouted, "it would be wrong to give him this terrible diagnosis!"

"You will kill him if you tell him!" his brother screamed.

In the feedback session afterward, the brother with the bloody forehead complimented me. "You were so calm!" he said. "I found it very challenging to scream at you."

Each week, someone from my POM small group would venture to the fake clinic to see a complicated patient. Because we were the bilingual POM group—some more bilingual than others—our encounters were made even more complicated by the fact that they were in Spanish.

After the feedback session, the student would be given a DVD recording of their encounter, and our small group would watch it together. To watch yourself, as a second-year medical student, stammer and blush through a half-hour Spanish encounter with an actor trained to deceive you about the problems he is having with his erections, is an experience so acutely humiliating that it should properly be undertaken only with copious amounts of gin. In those afternoon sessions where we watched one another on video, I was grateful for the bonds that were growing between my classmates and me. We were all pretty awkward, and some of us were hilariously easy to shock. But at least we were kind to one another.

POM WAS ALSO LACED with "clinical encounters": half-day sessions in which we poor inept junior students would shrug on our immaculate white coats and trot over to the hospital to meet up with an actual medical team. In these clinical encounters, we performed exams and took histories, but it was purely for our own education. Nothing we did actually contributed to patient care. This made the clinical encounters feel awkward: we were bothering a sick person with an exam that was, for them, unnecessary. Even so, patients were usually very generous with us.

I was seeing lots of patients at St. Vincent's, but the hospital felt different. The first floor was still being repaired from Ike, and so it had been converted into a maze of temporary walkways past demolished spaces where industrial fans hummed and men in construction hats worked away. The UTMB hospital complex would be confusing under the best of circumstances. It seems to defy physics. You turn a corner and suddenly find yourself in a totally different building, and somehow—mysteriously—you cannot reenter the previous building from this floor.

No matter which of the entrances to this complex I started through, I immediately became lost. To make matters worse, we would be told to report not to a numbered room but "to the IMC" or "to the NICU" or "to the cardiac care unit." I always felt embarrassed to admit how lost I was—I was in a white coat, right? I should know exactly where I'm going! When I finally found myself near where I was supposed to be, I would stand around looking panicked until somebody from the medical team took pity on me.

"POM student?" they would ask.

"Yes!" Thank god.

The clinical encounters were meant to get us a modicum of experience before we started our third-year hospital rotations. They also served the purpose of getting us excited about third year. At that time, anything seemed more exciting to me than another night of studying the sodium channels in the distal convoluted tubule of the kidney. So, the clinical encounters worked for me.

One of my very first encounters was on surgery. I was invited into the operating room for an hour to observe while a senior surgeon removed a patient's gallbladder. I got there after the surgery had begun, so I never saw the patient awake. But as soon as I entered the operating room—masked but unscrubbed, because I wouldn't be allowed anywhere near the surgical field—I felt that I had come into a holy space.

The room was square, and tiled. The overhead lights were dim, and people in light blue gowns and gloves, with masks over the bottom half of their faces and paper caps covering their hair, stood silently with their hands folded in front of them. (This, I would learn, is a way to make sure your gloved hands stay sterile.) In the center of the room, floodlights poured down over the body of a draped woman. Only the skin of her belly could be seen, and it was taut from the carbon dioxide that the surgeon had inflated it with. Through a tiny incision, he worked a camera into the woman's inflated belly.

"POM student?" the surgeon said, breaking the quiet.

"Yes," I said.

"Is this your first time in surgery?"

"Yes."

"Welcome. Don't touch anything."

"I won't. Thank you."

"I mean, do not touch *anything*."

"Got it," I said, suddenly feeling that somehow I was making a mistake by letting the bottoms of my feet touch the floor.

The lighted camera—called a laparoscope—was at the end of a long-handled tool. And as the surgeon worked his way in, images from inside the woman's body appeared on a screen beside the operating table. I realized that the overhead lights were dim so that we could see this screen. And the belly was inflated, also, so that we could see around inside.

"Make sure you can see this," the surgeon said to me, and I moved slightly for a better view.

The inside of this woman was nothing like what I had seen in anatomy lab. Her intestines were bright pink and slippery, and they moved rhythmically with the action of peristalsis. She was alive. I remember making the obvious—but still, in its way—astonishing observation that the inside of the body is not bloody. The blood is contained in veins and arteries, so if you enter the body carefully, you see the smooth, clean surfaces of human organs working as they should.

As per tradition, the surgeon decided to ask me a question. I was the junior trainee in the room, and so I was expected to answer anything. Knowing this was my first surgery, though, he tossed me an easy one.

"What's that?" he asked, as the camera turned toward a dark, shiny lump in the abdomen.

Suddenly, I was totally disoriented. What was that dark organ? I knew we were supposed to be taking out the gallbladder.

"Um, the gallbladder?"

"That's the liver," he said. Of course, the liver: the most obvious organ in the abdomen. He didn't ask me any more questions, apparently realizing it would be fruitless.

The surgery proceeded tidily, as the doctor trimmed carefully through the tissue that connects the gallbladder to the bottom of the liver. He worked entirely through tiny incisions in the belly, guided by the camera as he snipped and clipped away with long-handled tools. He clamped the artery that provides blood to the gallbladder, as well as the duct that carried bile from the gallbladder to the intestine. When he finally grasped the gallbladder itself and pulled it through the incision and out into the world of the operating room, that final motion was clean and bloodless.

There was the organ itself, shiny and purplish, smaller in real life than it had been on the screen. A surgical tech put it into a silver tray, then sliced it open lengthwise so I could see the stones hidden inside.

Back under the lights, air escaped from the woman's inflated belly as the surgeon removed his tools. He neatly sewed up the three small incisions. All that would be left for the world to see of our time inside this woman's body were three tiny scars.

POM TOOK ME, for the first time, into Hospital Galveston. UTMB students undergo security clearance and training for prison work during their first year. The training includes, among other things, an armed prison guard in uniform opening up a box full of ordinary items that had been weaponized by prisoners: pens filed into sharp points, plastic forks with razor blades attached, metal reflex hammers somehow sharpened to resemble ice picks. The handiwork is sophisticated, and the demonstration left us medical students impressed.

The guard was proud to say that no medical student had ever been harmed at the prison hospital—although one had been briefly taken hostage. If we were taken hostage, we were to keep quiet and let the guards handle it.

Although our orientation to the prison hospital did not include the history of medical care for Texas prisoners, I was aware of some of that. In 1976, the Supreme Court ruled that prisoners' access to medical care is protected by the Constitution. Technically, the judges wrote that "deliberate indifference to a prisoner's medical needs" constitutes a violation of his or her Eighth Amendment right to freedom from cruel and unusual punishment. The case—*Estelle v. Gamble*—actually came out of Texas. A prisoner named J. W. Gamble had been assigned to unload cotton bales from a truck, and he was crushed by a falling bale. His back pain after the accident was ignored, and he was even put in solitary confinement for refusing to work because of his pain.

For a while after 1976, the TDCJ continued to run its own prison medical care. UTMB was a marginal part of the system, seeing prison patients along with other patients at John Sealy Hospital. But in 1979, Judge William Wayne Justice ruled that medical conditions in Texas prisons were unconstitutionally bad. He ordered an overhaul of the state prison medical system. This led to Hospital Galveston being built, in 1983.

The War on Drugs began in the 1980s, and prison populations skyrocketed. The TDCJ medical system was struggling, and multiple lawsuits showed that Texas prisoners had been mistreated or their medical problems had been ignored. UTMB signed a contract with the state in 1994, formally taking over medical care for about 80 percent of Texas prisoners. This arrangement is called "Correctional Managed Care."

Correctional Managed Care has not been without its failings, the most notorious of which occurred at a private prison called Dawson. Dawson State Jail was a women's prison, and most of the women there were serving short sentences. At least three women—

Shebaa Green, Pamela Weathersby, and Ashleigh Parks—are reported to have died after their treatable medical conditions were ignored by guards. Another woman, Autumn Miller, went into premature labor while serving a yearlong sentence for violating probation. Miller was a mother of two, and she recognized the cramps when she went into labor. But the guards ignored her, tossing a menstrual pad into her cell. She gave birth to Gracie Miller on the toilet in her cell. Gracie was only twenty-six weeks along, and she died four days later.

The problems at Dawson were not with the medical care per se. In most cases, the problem seemed to be that guards were ignoring serious complaints instead of relaying them to the medical staff.

But the prisons are notoriously short on medical staff. A glance at the TDCJ unit directory shows, for example, that many units don't have twenty-four-hour medical care. A prison with thirteen hundred inmates averages eleven medical staff members. That number may include only one physician, with most staff being vocational nurses and medication aides. And prisoners are a bit more likely to be sick than your average Texan: not only do many come from poor backgrounds but the prisons have high rates of infectious diseases, including tuberculosis, HIV, and hepatitis C. The state is always trying to cut the cost of prison medical care, and UTMB struggles to keep up with the need, just like the TDCJ did in the eighties. In 2006, the chief of UTMB Correctional Managed Care told reporters that "Right now, the system is constitutional . . . but we're on a thin line."[*]

So it was with some trepidation that I took my first steps into the prison hospital. I knew I had a lot to learn in there, but I wasn't sure exactly what the lessons would be.

———

To get into the prison hospital as a provider, you take the elevator to the fourth floor of John Sealy Hospital. You walk down a normal hospital hallway and turn left. Then you push open a perfectly ordinary door marked "TDCJ," and you find yourself at the entrance to a maximum-security prison.

Before coming through this door, I had emptied my white coat of the usual tools, including my cell phone. All I had was my badge, a notebook, and a pen. The double door swung open to admit me into a small, rectangular space. Directly in front of me was a wall of bars with a gate in the middle. To my right there was a cabinet that held a few purses and sets of keys, and to my left, behind another wall of bars, a guard sat in front of a computer.

"Badge," he said.

I passed him my badge, which he ran through some kind of scanner. Then he looked at the computer to make sure I had security clearance.

"Empty your pockets," he said. I had only the paper and pen.

"No phone, right?" he asked.

"No phone," I said. In the early mornings, when a rush of physicians and nurses comes through, a second guard is on hand to search everyone. But I seemed to have missed that, and after handing my badge back to me, the guard pressed a button and the gate slowly opened.

I passed into a long hallway—the sky bridge that connects John Sealy to Hospital Galveston. There were no windows. A partition ran the length of the hallway at chest level, separating people going into the prison from those leaving. On the other side, an elderly man in white was being pushed in a wheelchair toward the gate I had come through. His lips sagged inward over a toothless mouth with no dentures. He was shackled at the wrists and ankles. Neither he nor the guard pushing his wheelchair looked up at me as I passed.

At the far end of the hallway, I waited for another gate of metal bars to buzz and open for me. Then I found myself truly in a prison for the first time. I was in a large room with barred, gated hallways leading off at angles. In the middle of the room was a guard stand, also surrounded by bars. From there, guards could watch all the gates as well as the elevators and the doors that led to the stairwell. I asked a guard how to get to my assigned unit, and she pointed me to the elevators marked "Staff Only." As I waited for my elevator, a guard pushed another man in a wheelchair out of the opposite elevators. This man was shackled with thick chains, and he had a mask over his face.

It was a relief to meet up with the medical team. They introduced me to the patient I was assigned to interview, leading me past the guard who watched the door to his room. He was a lower-security patient, so the guard didn't have to come into the room with me, but she watched us through the glass wall. All I had to do was take a thorough history, write my note, and I could go.

My patient was a Spanish-speaking man in his early forties. He was in the hospital because his heartbeat was irregular, and a cardiac monitor was strapped to his chest. He'd fainted in his cell a week ago, and he was transported to Hospital Galveston after getting emergency treatment at a local ER. The bus ride from his prison unit to Hospital Galveston had taken two days. I know that sounds improbable, but it's true—the buses stop at various prisons along the way, picking up and dropping off people. It takes a long time.

There was no chair in his room, so I stood a bit awkwardly looming over his bed. Even so, we fell easily into talking. He told me that his heart troubles had started the first year he was in prison, but that he was going to get out next year. "I am afraid, though," he said.

"Why are you afraid?"

"I want to be able to do things when they release me. And with my bad heart, I don't know if I'll be able to."

"What kinds of things do you want to do?" I asked.

"I want to climb mountains!"

This made me smile, but he was totally in earnest. My patient was not only an inmate of the state of Texas but also a potential mountaineer.

"What can I do now," he asked me, "to take care of my heart?" In the free world, this is a dream question. Doctors can seem like we're always nagging people about diet and exercise, but here was a forty-year-old patient who wanted to know what steps he could take to protect his heart so he could climb mountains! I was eager to help him out.

"Well," I said, "you want to take your medications if they prescribe them."

"Oh yes," he said.

"And aside from that, a healthy diet and exercise are good ways to take care of your heart."

His face fell. He explained that his access to space for exercise was very limited. "And the food in prison is very bad," he said. "I am sure that it's high in fat. It's just . . . It's very bad. I do not believe it is healthy for my heart."

"Oh," I said. There was nothing I could do about that; he was probably right about prison food not being the healthiest option. What else could I say, when my best advice was useless to him?

"I want you to climb mountains when you get out," I said, trying to console him. "I'll keep hoping for you."

"Thank you," he said.

When we were almost done with his history, a guard came into the room. It was time for my patient to go downstairs for cardioversion—a procedure where they use electric shocks to convert an irregular heartbeat into a normal one. I had never seen anything like that before, so I tagged along.

My patient was placed in a wheelchair and shackled at the wrists and ankles. The guard took him down the patient elevator, while I took the staff elevator. Then we passed separately back down the long hallway and into the regular hospital. The white-coated people passing in the hallway hardly glanced down at my patient, and I trailed behind the guard into another hospital room. There, my patient was moved onto a bed and shackled again. The guard waited close by.

A nurse stopped by the bed and swiftly placed an IV line in my patient's arm, saying nothing to him. She put some kind of medication in the IV.

"What is happening?" my patient asked me.

"Um, let me find out. I think they're going to shock your heart."

"To shock my heart?" he repeated, sounding terrified but also a little slow. The IV medication must have been a sedative.

"I mean, gently. So it returns to a usual rhythm." I tried to sound confident and calming, but the truth is I wasn't sure exactly what was happening. Nobody else in the room—a busy room with four beds separated by curtains, and doctors moving from bed to bed—spoke to my patient. Did anybody speak Spanish? Could they explain to me or him what was about to happen?

"Okay, let's go," a doctor said, having materialized at the bedside. He drew the curtains shut and began doing something to my patient, but my understanding of what was going on was very vague, and I could hardly see between the guard and the doctor. They must have given him another sedative, because my patient was asleep before his body jerked from the electric shock.

The doctor turned to the heart monitor, which began to show a normal rhythm. Then he moved away from the bed. The guard picked up a magazine. Everything, it seemed, was over.

I backed out of the room and hurried down the hall toward the hospital entrance. My note was written and my patient was asleep. I felt like there was nothing I could do for him—I couldn't insist that he get a better diet in prison, or help him find ways to exercise, or cure his underlying heart condition. I couldn't give him the freedom he needed to care for his illness, or ensure that he would have medical care once he got out of prison. All I could do was have a sort of human conversation with him, and hope that it mattered.

I know now that the care my first prison patient received—sedated cardioversion for an arrhythmia—was technically competent and appropriate for his condition. But without the human touches that I was learning to offer at St. Vincent's (or even the basic courtesy of explaining what we were doing to a patient's body), technically competent medical care could be a terrifying experience.

CHAPTER 8

ONE DAY IN APRIL WHEN THE ISLAND WAS BLANKETED IN fog, I went to neurobiology lab to dissect a human brain. The last hour was a slide show, running through slide after slide of dissected slices of brain. They all looked the same to me: gray and featureless, reduced. I needed to memorize their names and locations, their functions, the other brain structures in communication with each. *What are these structures?* I thought to myself. *This is nothing.* We replaced the brains in their vats, and I walked from campus toward my house. I was moving down an alley paved with broken oyster shells. I could hear the buzzing of the laboratory buildings, and my bag was heavy on my shoulder. *This is not a symptom of depression*, I realized. *This is who I am. I have always wanted to die.*

I know now that it was depression, the affliction that comes on about a third of medical students at some time. But then, I thought I had made a great realization. It was almost psychotic in its clarity, as when my schizophrenic patients would describe the moment they realized they were in fact telepathic, or would gaze out the window of the clinic and casually note the particular pigeon that was in fact an angel, bringing a message from God. It was more lucid than most of my moments: knowledge revealed, perfectly clear.

I got home, checked on my dog, and the message faded out a little bit. It grew less compelling, but it didn't go away. *This is not a symptom of depression. This is who I am.*

It had been a difficult semester. I'd had falling-outs with my two closest friends in medical school. Looking back, it's hard to know if we fell out because I was depressed, or if I was depressed because I didn't have my friends. We're all friends again, in the long run of things, but that spring was bad. I lived in a creaky second-story apartment of a Victorian house with my dog, who would balefully watch me study and, if he thought I couldn't see him, eat a shoe.

Charlie is a good dog, but he is not much for emotional cues. One day that April I was sitting on the edge of my bed crying, and Charlie came up and began licking my cheeks. *This is it*, I thought. *This is the breakthrough. He's trying to comfort me!* But then he got excited, and bit my face.

I was probably not very emotionally supportive to him at that time either, to be fair.

The apartment got pretty fetid. Galveston has a recycling center at the end of the island, and you have to drive down there to drop off your recycling. Like a good Austin gal, I aspired to recycle. But when I was depressed, the trip down the island became too much for me. So piles of newspaper, empty bottles, and half-washed cans of Ranch Style Beans built up in my kitchen, and roaches built up behind them. Margaret would come over occasionally, and—in a true act of kindness—take my recycling downstairs and throw it away.

I had gotten Charlie with a boyfriend (now defunct) and occasionally late at night when the conviction became too much for me—*I have always wanted to die*—I would walk over to the yellow house where my ex-boyfriend lived, and ask to come talk in his room a while. But sometime in April he told me that I was not welcome there unless I was willing to sleep with him, so I stopped going. Then the yellow house was no longer my territory, and I was more alone.

I was not actually (I say now) going to kill myself. I learned my lesson from Frank: It's cruel. But the simple fact that I wanted to, that I was perfectly convinced that not-life was preferable to life, itself depressed me. I failed a test, was late to class, and stopped caring what I looked like. And nobody noticed, because in medical school it is possible to be surrounded by people and remain truly alone.

THREE THINGS GOT ME THROUGH IT. To be perfectly honest, the first was cigarettes. Smoking was like scratching an itch, inviting a little death into me. It took the edge off, and after smoking a cigarette I would find that my mind had turned to some other preoccupation. I do not recommend smoking, of course, but I came to understand one reason why people do it.

The second thing was my brother. He has a way of appearing when I need him. (The "way" is by receiving my panicky, tearful phone calls, buying a thousand-dollar ticket to fly from Alaska to Texas, giving up a couple weeks of work, and installing himself on my couch.) He stayed through two of the worst weeks, quietly cooking Vietnamese food and hanging out with my neighbor, Alyssa.

The final thing, and the thing that actually saved me, was that the school year ended. The year ended, and I turned down a scholarship to go to Colombia and work with a family physician for a month. The professor who had recommended me for the scholarship was shocked when I told her. "You may never have a chance like this again," she said. "To go abroad with everything paid for. It's special."

But I knew I was in no place for that, and I think the decision I made was life affirming. Instead of going to Colombia, I cleaned my apartment as best I could and went to Chicago to stay for a month with my best friends Delaney and Ryan. We would cook together in the evenings, and I started writing again, resurrecting a children's book project I had begun before medical school. Gradually, I came back into myself. One night I told Delaney what I had realized about death—that my desire to die was durable, not a symptom of depression but a part of myself. She listened quietly, then said, "No. I don't think that's right."

Delaney had known me for many years. I started to insist, but when I reached down into myself to resurrect that conviction, it was gone.

I write about this here because I think it's important to share. Medical students and physicians have high rates of suicide. Male physicians are about 1.4 times more likely than their nonphysician counterparts to die by suicide, and female physicians are 2.3 times more likely.* Medical students and residents are particularly likely to be depressed; studies have found that as many as 30 percent of medical trainees may screen positive for depression on a questionnaire. But depression is not a thing that we like to discuss—at least not when it comes to ourselves.

To do so, in fact, makes us professionally vulnerable. When you apply for a medical license in some states, you have to report whether you've been under psychiatric care. If you've been on medications or been seeing a psychiatrist, this admission can delay your licensure. The reporting requirement is meant to protect patients from impaired physicians, but in fact, it works the other way: By discouraging us from seeking psychiatric care, it makes both us and our patients more vulnerable. It drives a suicide-prone population away from the help we may need.

WHILE I WAS IN CHICAGO, Alyssa went over to my apartment twice a week to water my plants. One day she texted me, "Who's taking the plants?" I told her that I didn't know, and she sent me pictures: the pots were still there, but my three small basil plants had disappeared.

The next week, my last plant—a three-foot-high pencil cactus— disappeared in the same way. It was a mystery. With the plants gone, Alyssa stopped going over.

When I got back from Chicago, the mystery was solved. I opened the door of my apartment to find that the place was absolutely cov-

---

* Matthew Goldman, Ravi Shah, and Carol Bernstein, "Depression and Suicide Among Physician Trainees: Recommendations for a National Response," *JAMA Psychiatry* 72, no. 5 (2015): 411–412.

ered in rat shit. I looked across the nasty floor, and over at the pot where my pencil cactus had stood. *My plants have been eaten by rats,* I realized.

The apartment smelled rank, and as I walked in I felt a wave of shame. I was back in Galveston, back in the lonely apartment where I had become so depressed. I was no longer a writer, but doomed to be a medical student. I seemed so successful on the outside, but I knew that I was a failure in the one way that mattered most to me as a human being, because I had given up on writing and myself. Now, a plague had come.

I put down my luggage and went straight to bed.

That night, I dreamed of Frank. I was back in the auditorium at Portland State, where our physics class had been. It was the first class I had returned to after he died, and I recognized my Portland friends in the seats. I went from friend to friend, saying hello, grabbing their hands, but they each turned away from me, silent. It was as if they could not see me. I went to sit in the back, and Frank was next to me. I realized why he was the only one who could see me. "How could you do this, Rachel?" he said. "You've made a horrible mistake."

I was awakened from my dream by a loud banging sound. I lay in my bed for a minute, and the banging did not recur. So I got up, because I had to go to the bathroom. I walked through the dark apartment to the kitchen, and when I got there I heard another loud bang. I reached toward the shelf where the light switch was. When it came on, three huge rats jumped off the shelf. As they went, they knocked another can off the shelf—*bang*. They ran into the bathroom.

Clearly, I could not go to the bathroom. So that is how I began my second year of medical school: barely recovered from depression, pissing in the kitchen sink of my rat-infested apartment.

The dream had done its work, however. Within two weeks, I left that apartment. I started classes again, and began going back to St. Vincent's. That was when I met Mr. Rose.

CHAPTER 9

AT OUR FIRST VISIT, I LISTENED TO MR. ROSE'S STORY-telling. He told how he had worked on cars, been on a ship in the Merchant Marines, and how his cousin's little baby was doing. My life, in comparison—my books, my short white coat, my bike commute from home to the library and back again—felt pretty dry. And anyway, there was plenty of time to talk with him. We sat in one of the exam rooms at St. Vincent's, hearing the thumps and shouts of a basketball game on the court outside the window as we talked.

I'd picked up Mr. Rose's chart because he was a first-time patient, and I knew I'd get to do a whole social history and family history and a complete physical. Doing those things is good practice, and you always learn a lot. I was a second-year medical student so I was short on information but long on time, and we could sit in the exam room for a solid hour and a half while Mr. Rose told me about his pain.

The pain was nonspecific—that is, it wasn't clearly coming from the liver, or the pancreas, or the stomach, or anywhere. He'd had a couple of tarry, black stools—an ominous finding that suggests bleeding in the stomach. And he'd had some constipation, and he felt as if food got stuck in his throat, and he had a few other symptoms. His eyes were yellow, and his urine stank. It seemed everything was wrong, but none of it pointed clearly to anything. I asked about general symptoms—fatigue or weight loss—and he said he wasn't sure about his weight, but he figured he'd lost some from not eating. He used to weigh four hundred pounds. Then he lost one hundred pounds in one year, his diabetes resolved, and he somehow slid off the patient list at UTMB. He hadn't seen a doctor since then—four years ago. Somebody at his sister's church recommended St. Vincent's.

So I did everything I knew how to do. I did a full physical exam, noting that his belly was taut with fluid. A swollen belly suggests liver problems, so I spent a while asking Mr. Rose about things that can lead to liver disease: IV drug use, foreign travel, sexual activity, and transfusions—all of which can put you at risk for a hepatitis virus. Other drugs, herbs, or medicines. And, of course, alcohol.

Mr. Rose wasn't much of a drinker. His father had been a lifetime alcoholic who died of cirrhosis of the liver, so he knew what that looked like. "I drink," he said, "but not like him." I pressed him on the issue, and he said he'd have two or three beers at a time, once or twice a week. But that was before the pain started. Since the pain began, he hadn't been drinking at all.

The physical exam was very thorough, because the doctor volunteering that day had told me, "This is your chance to learn. At St. Vincent's, you need to lay hands on every single patient. You're going to see things here you won't see anywhere else."

I laid my hands—the hands of a second-year medical student—on Mr. Rose. His belly was tender all over, but on the upper left side it was exquisitely tender. Pressing on it caused so much pain that he moaned and, as if involuntarily, pushed my hands away. So I didn't press too hard right there. I was too tender myself, at that time, to know that a doctor must steel herself to press the hardest exactly where it hurts.

I checked his blood sugar and his heart rate; I tapped out the span of his liver; I pressed on his ankles and looked at his palms. I took a sample of his blood for labs. It took me three tries with the needle and

I raised a bruise on his inner elbow, but he didn't complain. He just looked at me in that quizzical way, with one eyebrow up, and said, "Doc, you sure are a student."

On the scale in the hallway, Mr. Rose was shocked to note that he had lost twenty pounds.

"When did you last weigh yourself?" I asked. A month ago, he'd weighed himself on the scale at the liquor store. Now that caught my attention, because he'd told me he never drank much, and hadn't been drinking at all since the pain began. So I asked him again about drinking. And he said no, he just walked up there with his cousin, and they have a scale you can use for a quarter.

That is one of the moments I think back to, in trying to figure how this story went awry: Mr. Rose standing in the hallway in his socks, talking about the scale at the liquor store. When I reported to the attending, I mentioned it. It introduced a note of skepticism, a nail on which we could hang a little mistrust.

Rapid, unexplained weight loss is a very bad sign, and it should have made us suspect cancer. But in this particular case, the attending physician was led to suspect alcoholism, instead. The detail about the liquor store scale took on more meaning than the weight itself. Even at St. Vincent's, where our mission is to care for the uninsured, it so happens that medical providers can have a hard time trusting a homeless African American man—a *poor historian*—when he says he doesn't drink. Not to mention his swollen belly. Or the scale at the liquor store.

ON THAT FIRST VISIT, I made a mistake. Mr. Rose had said his urine stank. So a fourth-year medical student named Chandler, who was directing St. Vincent's, told me to get a urine sample and do a urine dip. And I did. A urine dip is the simplest of lab tests. I walked to our little hallway laboratory with the urine sample, and followed the instructions on the bottle of test strips: you dip one in the urine, let it sit for sixty seconds, and then compare the little colored boxes on the strip with the example boxes on the side of the bottle.

When I checked Mr. Rose's strip after sixty seconds, every single value was abnormal. The strip said there was blood in the urine, ketones, and protein, and the pH was wrong. Surely I had messed up this test? They couldn't *all* be abnormal. I wrote down the results, then poured out the rest of the sample.

It stank so badly that I retched over the sink.

And by the time I was describing Mr. Rose to the attending physician, I had forgotten about the messed-up urine sample. I was worried about the pain that had brought Mr. Rose to the clinic, and the exquisite tenderness of his belly. Then there were the black stools. And the fluid in his abdomen, the trouble swallowing, the yellow eyes. There was so much wrong with this patient that I was struggling to tell his story at all, and I forgot about the urine.

AFTER MY FIRST VISIT with Mr. Rose, I took him on as my patient. Attending doctors and the student directors were always backing me up, but I made sure to be present at every one of his appointments. So, I saw him every week for months. He seemed to get a little bit sicker every time, his belly more swollen or his pain worse, but there wasn't much we could do without the studies we needed to diagnose him. At one point we sent him to the ER at UTMB to see whether he could get admitted to the hospital, but they just told him it wasn't a proper emergency and sent him back to St. Vincent's. Although a 1986 law called EMTALA—the Emergency Medical Treatment and Labor Act—requires hospitals with emergency rooms to accept and stabilize patients with emergencies threatening life or limb, patients who are not actively dying may not be accepted. Mr. Rose was clearly sick, but he wasn't actively dying.

Our working diagnosis was still alcoholic cirrhosis of the liver. So I would ask about alcohol, trying to do what the doctor had recommended, and Mr. Rose would tell me again that he didn't drink. "Lord no, I am not drinking," he would say. "I can hardly eat my yogurt." I stopped asking after I finally felt too embarrassed to push the issue. I believed him.

And what about that pain? St. Vincent's had a policy of not prescribing narcotics, so those drugs were out. He couldn't take drugs like ibuprofen because we were worried about bleeding in his stomach. So we didn't do much, and when Mr. Rose quietly asked me if it was okay that he took his sister's Norco sometimes, I nodded yes and was grateful he had access to something. It hurt him to stand, to move, to walk.

When the new year of medical school began, my first course covered the heart. Listening closely to Mr. Rose's heart sounds, I picked up an abnormality: an S3, which sounds like an extra beat. It's a sign of fluid backing up, and overfilling the heart. "I think he has an S3," I said to the doctor.

When the doctor double checked and verified the S3, he was so proud of me that he gave me a high-five—right in front of Mr. Rose. Then he explained what the sound meant.

My next class was on the gastrointestinal system, and I learned all about the liver. I learned that, in patients like Mr. Rose, one important study to do is the peritoneal tap. The peritoneum is a thin layer of tissue inside the abdominal wall. In a peritoneal tap, we push a needle through the skin, muscle, and peritoneum to take a sample of the fluid from the belly. In Mr. Rose's case, the protein content of the fluid could have been analyzed to distinguish between cancer and diseases like cirrhosis.

I started hounding my professors in the halls of the medical school after the lecture. "I have this patient at St. Vincent's," I would say. "I think he needs a peritoneal tap." One professor agreed, but there wasn't much he could do. He'd never done a peritoneal tap at St. Vincent's, and he wasn't convinced it would be safe. What if the needle punctured a loop of Mr. Rose's intestine? Fecal matter would leak into his abdomen and cause an infection. If the needle hit a vessel that caused rapid bleeding, would we send Mr. Rose to UTMB in an ambulance? And if we did that, what would be the consequences for the clinic? Every procedure has risks, and nobody knew how much risk was acceptable to take at St. Vincent's.

So Mr. Rose just kept coming back, telling his stories, living with his pain. We got to know each other pretty well. I would wave to him when I came into the clinic. He always showed up early, so he would be seen in the first round of patients. And I always pulled his chart. He started calling me "Doc." I learned a lot from him, and he believed in me.

ONE EVENING IN EARLY NOVEMBER I opened an e-mail with the subject line "Your Patient." *My patient?* I thought. *I'm just a second-year student. I don't have any patients.*

The e-mail was from Chandler. She was training in the emergency room in John Sealy that night, and Mr. Rose had come in, desperately short of breath. Chandler and her team checked him into the hospital. They put him on an oxygen mask, took blood samples, and did a CT scan. The results of the CT scan were copied into her e-mail. I held my breath as I read them.

There was a huge mass on one of his kidneys. (Why did I never feel that? Was I too gentle with my abdominal exam?) There were masses in his liver and his lungs. There were small masses in his brain. It could be nothing but cancer, metastasized all over his body. It had been there when he first came to St. Vincent's, and it had been growing inside him through all the months that I had been trying to care for him.

After reading Chandler's e-mail, I immediately bicycled the five blocks from the house to the hospital. Chandler met me outside, and walked me up to Mr. Rose's room. "Well, obviously it's cancer," she told me as we walked. "But we don't know what kind yet. We'll do the biopsy tomorrow."

"Oh man," I said.

"Yeah," she said. "Rachel, I'm really sorry." I hadn't even realized how upset I was until she said that, and my eyes filled with tears.

Mr. Rose was in the Intermediate Care unit—the IMC—where critically ill patients who are not quite sick enough for intensive care go. Chandler asked if I was ready, then opened his door and said, "Look who's here to visit you!"

"Hey!" Mr. Rose called out. "There's my doctor!" He spread his arms, with an IV trailing from one wrist. I walked over to his bed and gave him a hug.

"I'll leave you two to catch up," Chandler said. And then, more quietly, she said to me "Let me know if you need anything."

Mr. Rose had the head of his hospital bed tilted up so he could watch TV, and there was a barely touched dinner tray on the silver table beside his bed. He was on a heart monitor that beeped quietly, and a thin plastic tube blew oxygen into his nostrils.

"Well, sit on down," he said, and I pulled up a chair beside his bed. And from there our conversation rambled, in and out of sentences that I can rebuild from memory and those that are lost now. I remember that the strange surroundings—the machines, the IVs, the nurses who came and went—made me feel shy. I still felt out of place in the hospital back then. I remember that he was ebullient when he first saw me, but his voice dropped later. He told me that he had been short of breath for days, but then tonight he couldn't breathe at all, and he felt like he was going to faint. And, well, he knew he was sick, but now they were telling him it was cancer.

"What else have they told you?" I asked. I wanted to know if he knew as much as I did. I did not want to break the bad news; I was not part of the team taking care of him in the hospital, and I didn't know all the details. I was just a second-year student.

"They don't really know," Mr. Rose said, "but they think it's coming from my kidney. Not my liver like that one doctor was saying."

"From the kidney," I repeated. And in that moment, sitting beside my first patient, a cold wave of recognition swept down through my body. Kidney cancer. The urine sample. It was cancer that caused his urine sample to be all wrong. That urine sample I had misunderstood, and then forgotten. I remembered it right then and fell silent, stunned by guilt.

"I'm so sorry," I finally said. I could not begin to say everything I was sorry for.

"Well, you know," he said, apparently trying to comfort me. "They're going to do some kind of a test tomorrow."

"A biopsy."

"Tomorrow," he said. "And it may turn out to be one of those real treatable kinds of cancers."

"Right," I said. But I didn't believe it—not when it had already spread so far.

"I'm waiting to call my brother until I know if this is really serious or not," he said.

I knew it was serious. But I held my silence, thinking that a second-year medical student should not interfere with the doctors on the hospital team. *They will tell him when the time is right*, I told myself.

We chatted for a while longer. When I stood up to leave, he said, "Well, now you know where I am. So you can come visit."

But I never did. I never had the courage to go back, and soon it was too late. Three months later, I read his obituary in the *Galveston County Daily News*.

TWO YEARS LATER, after my third year of medical school, I would find myself telling this story to a group of first-year students. It was in an afternoon seminar on the medical humanities led by Dr. Susan McCammon.

There were around fifteen of us in the room. We had gathered to read and discuss a poem, but somehow the conversation turned—as it does—to patients. And I began telling the story of Mr. Rose: How I forgot that urine sample, and we couldn't get him care, and he died. How he had asked me to be near him when he was in the hospital, but I felt so guilty about my mistake that I abandoned him. Telling the story, I was surprised to find myself crying. It is so rare, almost forbidden, to cry in front of other medical students.

"How do you wish it would have been different?" Susan asked me gently.

The answer to that question was so vast that I could hardly speak it: I wish Mr. Rose could have been insured. I wish he'd had a primary care doctor who caught his cancer early. I wish at least we could have gotten him the care he needed, even if it was too late to cure. I wish I had the power to do what I was supposed to do, and provide him with medical care. I wish my first patient, the first patient I loved, the first patient who trusted me, had lived. But how do you say all that when tears are still running down your face?

"I wish he could've gotten into the hospital sooner," I said.

Susan nodded. "And what do you wish you would have done differently?" she asked.

"Well, I wish I wouldn't have made a mistake," I said.

"We make mistakes," she said. "It happens to all of us."

And then I thought a little more. "I wish I had gone back to see him," I said. "Even though I made a mistake, and he was dying. I wish I had had the grace to stay by his side."

CHAPTER 10

THE LUNGS ARE EASY TO LISTEN TO. HEALTHY BREATH sounds are regular whooshes, as if the air were a faraway electric train passing sixteen times per minute. Fluid makes crackles: little pops when the air passes through a skein of water. Areas of no sound could mean a bad infection, or a growth, or a collapsed lung—depending on what else is going on with the patient. There are sounds called wheezes, rales, and rhonchi. By the Thanksgiving of my second year of medical school, I had listened to a hundred pairs of lungs, and I could pick up these abnormalities.

So what made me think that the most abnormal finding of all—a whole lung that made no sound—was normal? Maybe it was the way my grandmother's backbone, twisted to one side from scoliosis that was never treated, changed the landscape of her body. Or maybe it was just my own lack of experience.

I took the coast road from Galveston to Port Aransas that Thanksgiving. I drove the twenty miles down Galveston Island to its narrow southern end, where the San Luis Pass separates it from the next barrier island. The day was bright and cool, and pelicans flew low over the water. After Galveston and Surfside, I turned toward Freeport to drive through the industrial towns: refineries, ports, and more refineries loom along the Texas coast. When I was a kid, I thought the refineries at night looked magical, like glittering fairy castles with tongues of colored flame at the top. From Freeport I jagged inland through Brazoria County with its lush oaks, then farther south through coastal plain—a remnant of the warm shallow sea that covered Texas in Paleozoic times. Trilobites were abundant here. Two hundred and fifty million years later, native people gathered oysters and conch on the shoals that start to crop up after you cross the Copano Bay. Today, you could go there in a flat-bottom boat to hunt stone crabs at low tide.

Soon I was in the little shrimping towns, then skipping from island to island along a long causeway to Port Aransas. The sun gleamed off the bay and I saw fishermen out wading. The last step to Port Aransas is a five-minute ferry ride across the ship channel.

Things in town looked the same that Thanksgiving: the fake shark head at Dolphin Docks, the souvenir shops, the boats huddled in the harbor and the empty beach. It was cool and windy. My stethoscope dangled from the rearview mirror. Thanksgiving is a family holiday for Port Aransas, without the crazy influx of summer tourists. The grocery store closes Wednesday night, then you're on your own.

Port Aransas is a lot like Galveston, though much smaller, and the water is clearer. Habitat for birds and other wildlife in the surrounding bays and lagoons has been better protected. But if you look offshore from the beach at night, you can pick out the oil rigs from the tankers waiting to come into the ship channel by the way the oil rigs blink. Fish congregate around the rigs, which serve as a sort of artificial reef; anchor nearby and you might catch red snapper or even tuna. The health risks of living farther north on the Gulf Coast are well-known: The stretch of refineries along the Louisiana and Mississippi coasts form what's called a "cancer belt" for nearby residents, who die earlier than average, and from strange cancers. In Port Aransas, and on down toward Brownsville, the risk of living on the industrial coast is not well documented. We had to evacuate once in junior high, when a tanker carrying a chemical gas caught fire in the ship channel. Cars backed up on the long road down the island, and when the wind changed, the chemical blew over us where we were waiting in that line. My eyes watered a little bit, but nothing serious happened. Refineries have blown up in Corpus Christi and Texas City. But in Port Aransas, we feel pretty safe from all that.

We live on the road that goes straight from the ferry through the middle of town to the beach. There are three stoplights in Port Aransas now—there used to be only two, and the third one was the subject of much debate in the local newspaper. You go through two stoplights on the way to our house, and then a stop sign next to the Mustang Island RV Resort, where we lived when we first moved here in the summer of 1994.

My grandma was visiting that Thanksgiving of my second year of medical school. She had been a healthy lady in her seventies, except for the scoliosis. But this time she wasn't doing so well. She had a light but persistent cough that wouldn't go away. Then one night, the week before I came in, she had what seemed like a TIA—a transient ischemic attack—which is basically a ministroke that clears up quickly. She smacked her lips five times at the dinner table and her cheek drooped. Then it stopped. My parents made a phone call, and a local guy from the EMS came up the stairs in his uniform. He'd been in the class behind me in Port Aransas High School, and he knew my family.

"You can take her into the hospital," he said to my parents, "and they'll run all these tests. They'll scan her brain, and then they're going to tell you it was a TIA. There's not any treatment she needs right now. So, it's up to you."

My family stayed home.

Grandma was also having a hard time going up and down the stairs, especially the outside stairs from our first story down past the pilings to the ground. It would take her thirty minutes and she hated it; she moaned the whole way, so it was a small miracle that my mom got her to the doctor at all for her persistent cough. The cough didn't seem like much: soft but persistent, once or twice a minute, and grandma felt like she had something in her throat. She had a low fever that came and went, and the usual pain from her twisted back. When Mom took her in for the cough, the doctor didn't find anything.

We didn't have a doctor in Port Aransas the first years we were here. You still have to cross the causeway for a hospital. I went to the ER over the causeway in Aransas Pass one night with a kidney infection, and they had one doctor running the whole emergency room. Which is just to say, these towns are small. My graduating class was thirty-five kids.

Grandma was a farmer's daughter in rural Arkansas, and then a secretary and a farmer's wife. They either didn't catch her scoliosis until it was too late to treat it, or couldn't afford the treatment—back braces, surgeries that had a slim chance of succeeding if done after puberty. Treatments have improved since the 1940s, but scoliosis is still common.

She was tall like me, and she was beautiful. After high school, she went to Lincoln for secretarial school, cooking for a family there in exchange for room and board. Her aunts told her she was an old maid at twenty, but then she met my grandfather at a sing: all the Ozark families would come together in a church to sing. They'd call all the women up to sing a hymn, then everybody related to so-and-so, then all the mothers, the fathers, the oldest children. Grandma had a beautiful voice that she did not pass along, but both my mother and I have her middle name: Great-grandmother Ora Mae, Grandma Lena Mae, my mother Reta Mae, and me. It's an old-fashioned name now, Southern and rural. I'll give it to my daughter, if I have one.

As Grandma got up into her seventies, her spine twisted into a bent S, humped up, and ached. She walked with a cane, and would threaten to whack us with it but never did. (She also threatened to whack George W. Bush, Saddam Hussein, and preachers who spend too much time trying to raise money during a sermon.) But by Thanksgiving she was hardly walking at all. I would rub capsaicin cream on her back for the pain, and slept beside her some nights for company.

They say you shouldn't treat your family, and I know that's right. In Grandma's case, it went like this: After the cough didn't go away, her pain was so bad that she didn't want to leave the house again to go to the doctor. My mother was afraid of pneumonia, so she asked me to listen to grandma's lungs. I pulled up her shirt in the back. On her left side, there was the regular whooshing of breath, clear all over with no fluid. On the right side, I heard nothing. Her back sounded dull on the right side wherever I tapped, instead of hollow like a normal lung field. Her spine was twisted over that direction; I thought maybe I just couldn't hear through the bone and muscles. I didn't listen in the front, too shy to ask my grandmother to pull her shirt up over her breasts.

"I don't hear any fluid," I said to my mother in the kitchen. "I don't think she's got pneumonia."

We baked four pies—apple, cherry, and two pecan—and my grandmother came out to sit in the recliner for Thanksgiving dinner.

WHEN I CAME BACK three weeks later for Christmas, everything was worse. The pain was worse, and she seemed confused. Even getting across the hall to the bathroom was an ordeal. She was repeating weird sentences—"Holy moly macaroni rack"—and for the first time in my life I saw her get really angry.

One night when I was lying in the bedroom with her, she asked me if I thought she was dying. I don't know why she asked her granddaughter this. Maybe because I was in medical school, or maybe she was just confused and it was late.

"Oh, Grandma, you're not that old," I said. "You could live for a long time."

"Oh, Lord," she replied. "I hope not."

AFTER CHRISTMAS WE CANCELED her flight back to Arkansas. Mom rented a car, and she and my brother drove Grandma to Springdale. She suffered on the way, and they went straight to the hospital; my uncles and cousins met them there.

It wasn't scoliosis that had prevented me from hearing air moving on her right side. I might have figured that out if I had listened in the front. I might have thought twice if I knew more, if I wasn't just a student, or if I loved my grandmother less and could have thought clearly through what was right in front of me.

Her whole lung was obliterated by cancer. It was in her brain—*that drooping lip, those weird phrases she was repeating*—and her bones—*that pain.*

When I think about it now, there are so many things that complicate this story. I think about that small-town EMS guy who cared about my family, who couldn't have had the medical training to know that what seemed like a TIA was actually from cancer working its way into her brain. I think about how her scoliosis was never treated, so the pain seemed almost normal. Her body was marked by that untreated disease, twisted and bent, and it confused me. And then there's me: a second-year medical student, too inexperienced to even know how little I knew.

She went straight into hospice. My mother never left her side. I drove up for the last few days, with Charlie. We slept overnight in my car at a Walmart parking lot in Oklahoma; Charlie would pop up from time to time to growl at the semitrucks that rumbled past on the highway.

We made it to Springdale the next morning. Grandma was in a residential hospice facility. She squeezed my hand when I got there, but her last words had already been spoken. Over the next few days, I would sit in the room with her and my parents and family, and step out sometimes to study or talk with cousins.

Sometimes, I would lay my face on her chest to listen to her breathing. Her breath was regular for days, and then it grew ragged. There was no sound of breathing on the right, where the cancer had choked out her whole lung—just the thrill of her heart. I felt like I was already a different person then: a medical person, who would experience this death in a different way.

One afternoon in the hospice facility, my uncle asked me what exactly was happening with her body, since she wasn't taking food or water. I knew how to answer that question.

"When people who are dying stop eating and drinking," I said, "their body doesn't want food. The gut kind of shuts down. Everything shuts down gradually. Pretty soon she'll stop making urine, and then her heart will slow down and she'll pass away."

She died after dozens of visitors, with us all around her telling stories and praying.

After she passed away, a nurse came into the room. She listened to my grandmother's heart, and listened to her lungs. Everything was quiet.

CHAPTER 11

JANUARY ON GALVESTON ISLAND BRINGS QUIET BEACHES, migratory white pelicans, and the MUTA-GTA: male urogenital teaching assistants/gynecological teaching assistants. The MUTA-GTA (pronounced "moota gouda") is a gathering in which second-year students are taught to do breast and genital exams. For a few students, the MUTA-GTA is the first time they've touched the real live genitals of another human being. For many, it's the first time they put a finger into a man's anus. For all, it's quite an experience.

My group gathered in the standardized patient lab—a medical theater designed to look like a clinic—in the afternoon. The MUTA-GTA is a bit different from other SP experiences. For this most sensitive exam, the patients actually teach as you go. They're paid well, and they want to make sure student doctors learn to do these exams right.

After a brief introduction from our professor—the kind of doctor who is so precise and so socially awkward that you can't help but trust him—we went in groups of three into the patient rooms. My group consisted of two guys, and me.

"Now, y'all wash your hands!" the woman awaiting us called out. "I don't want y'all even coming anywhere near me till y'all wash your hands!" So we washed our hands, one after the other, and then gathered around the end of the exam table in a huddle. Our patient was sitting on the table, dressed in a gown with a sheet over her legs. We introduced ourselves.

"All right, now I know they've told y'all what to do, but I'm just gonna walk you through it. Okay?"

Okay.

"So, we're going to start with the breasts. Now don't go asking me to lay down. You just want me to start off sitting right here and taking the gown down so you can look at the breasts."

"Um, yes ma'am," I said.

"Now you ask me if it's okay to untie my gown in the back."

"Is it okay if I untie your gown in the back?"

"Go ahead," she said.

I untied her gown, and then she lowered it so she was naked from head to waist.

"All right now. You want me to hold my hands up behind my head like this, with my elbows out, and you just look at the breasts. What are y'all looking for?"

"Um, abnormalities," the student to my left said.

"Okay, like what? Don't just tell me 'abnormalities.'"

We started listing them: differences in size or shape. Scars. Dimpling of the skin. Retracted nipples. Redness.

"Good, now do y'all see anything like that?" We did not.

"So, you just say that my breasts look 'normal.' Don't go saying they look 'great,' or 'awesome,' or anything like that. Say 'normal.'"

"Your breasts look normal," one of the guys said, blushing deeply.

"Okay, now you're ready to do the breast exam. So, pull out my footrest."

One of the guys pulled out the footrest at the end of the bed, and our patient laid down on her back. "Now, you want to make sure I am as covered as possible at all times, right? So don't go leaving me with both of my breasts hanging out. Use your drape! Who's going first?"

I was designated to go first, because I'm a woman.

"Rub your hands together!" the patient said. "Don't go touching me with those cold hands. Brrrr." So I did, and then I started the exam, with me telling her what I was doing and her calling out instructions. "Really get in there and feel, now! If I have a lump, I sure want you to find it so don't be skimping on me. And get up in my armpit, too, because you know there's lymphatic tissue up there."

"Yes, ma'am," I said. I was pressing my fingers into her breasts, trying to feel all the way through the tissue to her chest wall.

"You ain't gonna hurt me."

"Okay."

"Now, what's the thing that tells you that you've done a thorough breast exam?" she asked.

"Um, time."

"That's right! You want to spend at least four minutes! Now that's going to feel like a long time, but you need to do it because I want to know you're being thorough. So take your time."

"Yes, ma'am," I said.

"Now, you can start on the other breast," she called to one of the guys. After we had all had a turn, she sat up again and one of the guys retied her gown.

"Now it's time for the vaginal exam," she said. "Gloves on! The first thing you need to know, is *be gentle.* You don't want to go leaping into anybody's vagina like some kind of cowboy. You go slow, and you be respectful."

"Yes, ma'am," one of the guys said.

"Before you even touch me at all, you want to make sure I'm doing okay. Am I right?"

"Yes, ma'am."

"That's right." And she walked us through it, starting with the bimanual exam, where you put two fingers into the vagina to feel for the cervix, then run your hand over the belly to feel for the uterus and ovaries. "Use plenty of lube!" she said. "And don't just surprise me by putting your fingers into my vagina. You tell me I'm going to feel the back of your hand on the inside of my leg, and then I'm going to feel your hand on my vulva. Am I right?" she called down from the end of the table.

"Yes, ma'am."

"I don't feel any ovaries," one guy said.

"That's all right," she said. "They're in there. You can't really feel them a lot of times when they're normal. You just keep practicing and you'll get it."

Finally, it was on to the cervical exam. "Now you want to use both those packets of lube," she said. "And you put that speculum in sideways, not like it's going to be when it's open. Put it in sideways, then you turn it and open it up once it's in there."

Magically, like the easiest thing in the world, her cervix popped into view at the end of the speculum.

"Hey, there it is!" one guy called out. "I can see your cervix!"

"Nice!" she said.

A FEW WEEKS AFTER THE MUTA-GTA, I was waiting to register my car at the DMV and got to talking to the woman next to me. She was a nurse practitioner who specialized in gynecology at a private clinic on the mainland.

"Oh, interesting!" I said. "I just got trained to do speculum exams."

"That's great," she said. "How many have you done?"

"Just the one, so far, in training," I said.

"Well, you'll get it," she said. "Don't worry. I take students in my clinic sometimes, but I don't let them touch my patients until they've spent a week at the prison clinic. You go there, and you can do twenty pap smears in a day."

"I see," I said. It was a simple calculus: in a week, you'd do a hundred pap smears. So before touching the genitals of an insured woman, a student needed to practice on a hundred poor women. I knew on some level that medical training worked like that, but it was strange to hear it said aloud so uncritically.

But as it turned out, my training would be just like that.

———

After the MUTA-GTA, I started doing speculum exams at St. Vincent's. I had already observed a few, and finally an upper-level student turned to me in the hallway outside a patient's room and said, "Why don't you lead this one? I'll watch you."

So I led the encounter. The patient was a twenty-six-year-old mother who needed a routine pap smear. She was a Spanish speaker, and very quiet. She moved her head "yes" or "no" to answer most of my questions. Then when I asked her to undress while we left the room, she lowered her eyes and nodded. Her hands were gripping her purse.

I stepped out along with the senior student, and we waited for a minute in the hall. "She seems really nervous," I said. "Are you sure I should do this one?"

"You can do it," he said. "You've done the MUTA-GTA, right?"

"Yeah."

"So it's time. See one, do one, teach one, right? I'll be there if you need anything."

So I nodded, and we knocked on the door to reenter our patient's room.

Inside, she was sitting on the end of the bed, with the sheet draped over her legs. Her face was tight with worry.

"Are you ready?" I asked. Silently again, she nodded. "Okay, go ahead and lie back, and I'll help you get your feet in the stirrups." She did, and I got into position with the senior student by my side. With the drape covering her knees, I could no longer see her face. I got the speculum and sample kit out from the drawer at the end of the bed, and began. Remembering what the MUTA-GTA patient had taught me, I said, "Okay, you're going to feel my hand on your leg."

When I touched her skin, she gasped. The senior student squeezed lubricant onto my fingers for the bimanual exam, and I felt her cervix at the back of her vagina, angling down from the top. I couldn't feel her ovaries, but her uterus felt small and normal. When that was done, the senior student handed me the speculum and nodded to me.

"You doing okay?" I asked the patient, and she replied with a barely audible "Yes." My hand was shaking with nervousness. I did not want to hurt this woman; I did not want to mess this up. I told her about each step I was taking, but she did not speak again.

It took me a couple of tries to find the cervix. I had to move the speculum around inside her, and I heard her gasp again. Then finally it popped into view, and I moved as quickly as I could to get the smear to screen her for cancer. When it was over, I said, "Okay, you're done." I breathed a huge sigh of relief, and helped our patient move her feet out of the stirrups. I felt a brief moment of triumph: I had done my first real pap smear. It didn't go perfectly, but it went fine.

Then I looked at her. Her hands were gripping the sides of the bed, and her face was turned to one side. She was crying.

"Oh my god," I said. "I'm so sorry. Did I hurt you?"

She shook her head and drew in a long, shuddering breath.

"I'm so sorry," I said again.

"No, doctor," she said. "You didn't hurt me."

"Are you okay?"

She nodded, and wiped the tears off of her cheek. "Yes, yes, I'm okay," she said. "Thank you, doctor."

The senior student and I stepped out again, and I turned to him. "That was nothing like the MUTA-GTA," I said.

"Yeah," he said. "It never is."

CHAPTER 12

AFTER I FINISHED MY SECOND YEAR, IT WAS TIME TO begin hospital training. I chose to move from Galveston to Austin for my third year of medical school, to train in the public hospital in downtown Austin. It was hard to leave St. Vincent's, but I knew I would be back after a year.

Training in Austin would give me a chance to see a different system: a truly public hospital, where the county indigent care program makes sure that most people can get adequate medical care.

The public hospital in Austin is a ramshackle hospital that the city always seemed on the verge of knocking down. The corridors are windowless and rambling; the scrubs are dispensed in a basement room that nobody can find, and you often walk into your patient's room to find a plumber working on the sink. It is, however, public: Everybody who came in was treated, and if they couldn't pay, social workers would get them registered for Medicaid or the county health care program, called the Medical Assistance Program, or MAP. MAP doesn't screen for citizenship, so even undocumented patients could get hooked up with hospital care and consistent primary care.

Along with two friends from college, I found a house within biking distance of the hospital. I moved my Labrador in and chose the sunniest room for us. Then, on a Monday in early June, I wandered the hospital basement for thirty minutes, collected five pairs of scrubs, and got ready to start my first real hospital rotation: three months of general surgery.

The fourth-year medical students prepared us poor third-years for surgery at orientation that afternoon. A tiny, peppy fourth-year stood before us and explained that we needed to be ready to answer a question from the doctors at any time. This is an old tradition in medicine, called "pimping."

"Get ready!" the fourth-year said. "The surgeons are going to pimp you execution style!"

"Execution style?" somebody asked.

"Yeah!" she chirped. "Like a firing squad!" She was going into surgery herself, and she seemed to think this was a very delightful way to be questioned.

"What do you mean, like a firing squad?" I asked.

"I mean, they line you up and ask the first student a question until he gets one wrong. Then, boom, he's dead! They move on to the next student, then the next, until everybody is dead."

"The surgeons can't actually execute us," somebody ventured.

"Oh, I don't know about that," the fourth-year said. "Every surgeon kills somebody sometime. Who knows? Maybe it could be you!"

Another fourth-year talked to us about volunteering at the Austin student-run free clinic, which sounded way smaller than St. Vincent's. It operates once every other week, and most of the patients get transferred out to regular primary care clinics. The students do acute stuff—lots of wound care for the homeless, for example—but they clearly weren't managing any cancer patients. That sounded pretty nice to me.

I'll learn how to be a doctor in a place with real access to care, I said to myself. There would be no more of the kinds of conversations I'd had with Mr. Rose. I wouldn't have to say, "You need a CT scan, but there's no way to get it." Access to care, I figured, would save both my patients and me.

———

THE FIRST SURGERY I scrubbed in for was an inglorious affair: it was a surgery to cut open and drain a perirectal abscess on a homeless man's inner buttock. Homeless people get skin infections a lot, because it's hard to wash your body or your clothes or your blankets when you don't have a home. In those conditions, any little cut or scrape can turn into a staph infection. I had seen a fair number of skin infections at St. Vincent's, but never one that required surgery.

The patient—let's call him Mr. Barnes—was already half-sedated by the time I met him in the preoperative holding room. I found his bed and introduced myself as the anesthesiologists were leaving. "Hi, Mr. Barnes," I said. "I'm Rachel. I'm a third-year medical student and I'll be assisting in your surgery today."

"Jesus Christ," he mumbled. "You're not going to do it, are you?"

"Uh, no," I said. "The surgeons are going to do it. I just stand there, I think."

"You think?" he asked, lifting his lip. "Is this your first fucking surgery or something?"

"Um, yes, actually, it is."

"Don't fucking touch me then," he said, and fell asleep.

For the record, I didn't perform surgery on Mr. Barnes. I followed him into the operating room, then stepped out to scrub my hands and get ready. The scrubbing is a complicated affair that takes ten minutes, a special brush, and two kinds of soap. Once you're scrubbed, you back through the door of the operating room, holding your hands out in front of you so you don't touch any surface. Then, a scrub nurse helps you get your gown and gloves on.

Once your gloves are on, your hands are sterile. This makes it possible to put your gloved hand into the open abdomen of a patient without introducing any bacteria. But you must not unsterilize yourself. If you touch your gown below the waist, or your glasses, or your mask, or anything that is not sterile, then your hands are unsterile and you get barked at by the scrub tech, regloved, and potentially ejected from the surgery altogether.

As I got more comfortable in the operating room, I was able to help with small tasks: reaching up to adjust the lights (which have handles covered by sterile slips), or using the sucking machine to suck blood up out of wounds when the surgeon shouts, "Suction!" Eventually I was allowed to sew up some wounds, and once, I cut off a toe. But in my very first surgery, I just kept quiet and tried not to touch anything. I did not, for example, touch Mr. Barnes.

EVEN SO, HE BECAME MY PATIENT. This meant that, during his recovery in the hospital, I would wake him up at 5:15 every morning to look at his buttock. He would greet me with a bleary "What the fuck are you doing here?" and I would explain that I was here to check his wound. Eventually he got used to me, and even started making some unwanted sexual comments.

One afternoon, I came into his room and he was on the phone. "I'm calling a goddamn lawyer right now so I can sue all you fuckers for malpractice," he explained to me.

"Okay," I said. "Have you had a bowel movement?"

"You'll all be fucking sorry," he said. "And no, I haven't had a bowel movement." He spoke the words "had a bowel movement" in a high, whiny voice, meant to make me sound ridiculous. It occurred to me that it actually was pretty ridiculous to say "bowel movement" to somebody who used the word "fucking" in almost every sentence. Maybe Mr. Barnes would trust me more if I just said, "Have you shit?" but I couldn't bring myself to do it.

"Any fever?" I asked.

"No," he said.

"Are you on hold?" I asked.

"Yes," he said.

"Good luck with the lawsuit," I said.

"Get out of my fucking face," he said.

"Okay! I'll be back with the rest of the team in about an hour."

"Don't you want to look at my asshole?" he asked. "You always want to look at my asshole."

"Not right now," I said.

"Oh, so my asshole's not special any more is it? Fuck you."

"It's still, um, very special," I said. "We just checked it already this morning, and you don't have any fever, so you're good."

"Go to hell, then, you fucking vampire pervert."

"Cheers."

Mr. Barnes was discharged after four days in the hospital, and I have not seen him since. His lawsuit, apparently, came to nothing. But his asshole healed.

ON SURGERY, WE STUDENTS TOOK Q-4 CALL. This means that, every fourth morning, we would find the most exhausted-looking student in the hospital, take the trauma pager from him or her, and prepare for a twenty-four-hour shift on the trauma team. If the beeper went off, it meant that the EMS was bringing someone into the hospital with trauma: a gunshot wound, a car wreck, the occasional stabbing. So everybody on the trauma team—a head surgeon, a resident, an intern, and a student—would run from wherever they were in the hospital out to the emergency room and get ready to receive the patient.

My first twenty-four-hour shift was led by the fearsome Dr. McAllison, a former Army surgeon. He preyed on the timid, and we learned quickly to answer his questions in an authoritative voice, even if we didn't know the answer. By day three of my surgery rotation, I could throw back my shoulders and proclaim, "I don't know, sir," with the best of them. What I lacked in knowledge, I was making up for in confident tones of voice.

I was on noon rounds with my team, standing outside a patient's room going over the differential diagnosis for abdominal pain, when the pager went off. Everyone stared at me.

I stared back.

Then I looked down at my pager. Then I looked back at the team.

"Rachel, you're being paged," the intern said.

"Oh my god," I said. "Should I go?"

"Yes, Rachel," the intern said gently. "That's what the trauma pager means. When it goes off, you go to the emergency room."

"Right!" I said. I was still standing there.

"So, go," the intern said.

"Right!" I turned around, with one last glance back at my team.

"Run," the intern said. I ran.

I burst into the emergency room, clutching the jangling pockets of my white coat, and found the rest of the team waiting outside a trauma bay. The patient hadn't arrived yet. I ditched my white coat in the nurses' station and, with the rest of the team, slipped on a yellow cloth gown and a plastic face mask—to protect myself from blood or whatever else might spray from the patient. All we knew about the patient was on the screen of the pager: she was an eighty-four-year-old woman who had been a passenger in a car wreck, wearing a seat belt, and she was barely conscious. Her blood pressure was low.

There was a long moment of silence. Then, down the hall, we heard the ER doors swing open as the EMS pushed the woman in on a gurney. They wheeled her straight into the trauma bay and the team swung into action. Somebody pressed a pair of shears into my hand and told me to cut off her clothes. "Expose!" the attending yelled, and I sheared right through her bra and panties so that all her clothes fell off beside her. There was a huge bruise on her belly—"seat-belt sign." When you see that, you worry about a lacerated liver or a ruptured spleen. I stood back while the team swarmed around her: checking her body for a source of bleeding, trying to start a peripheral IV, hooking her up to a heart monitor. The resident got an ultrasound machine and started looking inside her abdomen for pools of blood. Her pulse was weak and her blood pressure was dropping, so we knew she was bleeding somewhere inside.

"Hang two units of O negative," the attending said. Somebody ran out to get blood for a transfusion.

"Peripheral pulses not palpable," a nurse said. Her blood pressure had dropped so low that we couldn't feel her pulse in her arms or legs.

"I can't get a line in," the intern said.

"I'm trying on the other side, no access," the resident said. The woman was still breathing on her own, but nobody could manage to get an IV into her veins. Her veins were collapsing as she bled out into her own abdomen, and the IV just wouldn't go in.

"I'm going for a femoral stick," the resident said.

"Let's get to the OR," the attending said.

"Who are you?" a nurse said. And in that moment the attention in the trauma bay swung from the patient to a thin woman standing by the door, holding a purse. "Are you her family?" the nurse asked.

"No," the woman said. And I was quietly grateful, because I would not want this cutting off of clothes or digging for veins to be witnessed by our patient's child. "I'm the social worker. Her family is in the emergency room, and they want you to know she's DNR."

The tension in the trauma bay slackened. DNR means "Do not resuscitate." It meant, in this case, that we would not be going to the operating room. We would not slice this eighty-four-year-old woman's belly open to find and stop the bleeding inside, or transfer her to the ICU with a tube down her throat. It meant that, if she was dying, she was going to die.

Then the strangest thing happened. Most of the trauma team just wandered away. The social worker stayed, watching, in a corner of the room. The attending and the intern stayed, too. It was just the four of us, and we were all quiet. I watched as they tried over and over again to get an IV into her veins to transfuse blood. They went for the femoral vein, a big vein on the inside of the hip. And no luck. They tried using the ultrasound, and cutting open her leg to expose a vein. They were still digging around in her veins, cursing quietly, when the heart monitor began to slow.

"No chest compressions?" the intern asked.

"No," the attending said.

And then the lady started to die. She just bled out right there in the trauma bay, with two doctors poking uselessly at her collapsing veins. I couldn't believe it. You don't just die, in the hospital like that, from something so simple as bleeding. Right? You don't just die because we can't get a needle into your vein?

"All right, that's it," the attending said. And then everybody put down their instruments, tore off their yellow gowns, and walked away. The heart monitor was still beeping, but more and more slowly. I went to the door of the trauma bay and stood next to the intern. He seemed to think there was nothing more for us to do, so I also did nothing. He and the attending started talking about another case scheduled in the operating room, and the beeping of the heart monitor got even slower and less regular.

I knew that the woman was dying. *Should I hold her hand?* I thought. *Should I comfort her?* But I didn't. I stood silently with the rest of my team, thinking I would learn from them to do what a doctor does when someone dies.

The lesson I learned that day was that a doctor's work is done when there are no more interventions to do. We stood, speaking lightly of other things, in the door of the trauma bay. The only thing that marked our patient's death was the long slowing, and stopping, of the heart monitor's beep. Finally, our patient lay alone, naked, dead on the emergency room bed. She was eighty-four years old. This whole time, nobody had spoken her name. *That's it?* I thought. *That's it?*

The social worker came in and covered the body. She drew the curtains on the trauma bay so we could no longer see in. She must have cleaned up the body and the bay, because a few minutes later I saw her leading a middle-aged man and woman into the room. The woman clutched the man's arm, and drew her breath in sharply as the social worker pulled the curtain aside for them to step into the room where our patient's body lay.

I stood in the noisy ER hallway, barely hearing as the intern joked with a nurse. This was the first patient I had seen die. Guilt washed over me: I was only a medical student, but I was also a twenty-eight-year-old woman. I had loved my grandmothers. I knew better than to step away and let an elderly woman die alone.

I could have walked away from my team and to her bedside, and held her hand as she passed. I could have done anything at all. But I didn't. I just played the role I was being taught, instead of acting like a decent human being.

I WAS STILL FEELING SHAKEN as I hurried away from the ER, but there was no time to really calm myself. I was scheduled to assist on a lumpectomy in the operating room. I had not met the patient yet; I just knew that she had breast cancer and that we were doing a surgery to remove the cancer.

I rushed into the OR changing room, ditched my white coat again and slipped on a scrub hat, mask, and booties. My patient had already been brought back to the operating room, which meant that I was committing the cardinal medical student sin of being late to a surgery. I had missed my chance to place a catheter or help the anesthesiologist put a breathing tube down her throat. At this point I could not be helpful, but rather a distraction and an irritation to the surgical team.

As I scrubbed my hands and arms, I frantically reviewed what I knew about breast cancer. The attending was going to ask me questions, and I had not had time to review before the surgery. *Tumor, nodes, metastases,* I thought. *A mastectomy followed by chemotherapy and radiation. Routine breast self-exam is no longer recommended by the American College of Obstetricians and Gynecologists. Most patients diagnosed with this disease will ultimately die of it, even if they go into remission. Five-year survival rates of . . .*

I finished scrubbing and backed into the operating room as quietly as I could. As the door swung open, the surgeon glanced at me. I could feel her irritation. Any intrusion into the operating room is not only a distraction but also a potential source of contamination. Would the air blowing over our patient's body from the open door carry germs that would cause an infection? Would I de-sterilize something? The surgeon's brow furrowed, but her mouth was covered by the mask.

I walked over to the scrub nurse, who quickly gowned me and watched carefully as I put on my own gloves. My back was to the patient. I opened the sterile gloves and lay them inside their sterile paper packaging. I managed to get one glove halfway on, but fumbled with the second.

"Do it again, they're contaminated," the nurse said.

I cursed silently and then opened another pair of gloves. This time I managed to slip them over my hands in the proper fashion, without touching the outside of either glove with my hand. I was sterile and gowned.

I turned to join the operation, and that's when I saw our patient. She was not older than me.

She lay perfectly silent and perfectly still as the light poured down over her. Underneath the blue sterile drapes, I could see the side of one of her legs exposed in the light. It had the firm lean muscles of a bicycle commuter and, curving up her leg from the outside of her knee almost to her hip was a tattoo of a bird. An egret, I think.

I stood in that quiet space while the surgeon worked on her, quickly cutting through skin and dissecting down to her breast tissue. She removed a lump of breast, put one stitch in the top of the lump and one on the right so we could tell which side had been facing up inside the patient, and placed it in a sterile tray to be examined by the pathologist. If the margins were clear—that is, if no cancer cells were found at the edges of the lump—this young woman would go on through the rest of her treatment, and eventually have her breast reconstructed by another surgeon.

And yet she would likely die of it, soon or eventually. I knew that.

I had memorized that fact. Did she know, or did she want to know? I imagined her bicycling along the same route I took to the hospital, how her legs would flash in the sunshine for as long as she was as young and as alive as I was. The surgeon closed the wound with tiny stitches that ran up the edge of our patient's chest. I kept my folded hands to myself, and helped clean up when the surgery was over.

CHAPTER 13

I SAW DAMIEN'S X-RAY BEFORE I MET HIM. IN THE EMER-gency room hallway, looking at the computer screen that showed the results of his X-ray, he was just another diabetic foot. "What do you see?" my resident asked me.

"Osteomyelitis," I said. "There," pointing at a shadowy spot in the middle of the foot, where infection was eating away at the bone.

"Good," she said. It was unusual to get more than four or five words at a time out of a surgeon. I stared at the X-ray and kept quiet. At that time, I didn't mind that the surgeons didn't talk to us students or try to get to know us. They could be scary—I had seen several of them scream—and it seemed like we students were safer if the surgeons didn't know anything about us, anyway. Later, I would be on teams where I would be truly included in patient care and able to contribute, and I would realize how strange and dehumanizing the surgery experience was. But at the time, it was all I knew of the wards.

This was my next-to-last night of trauma call. By then, I'd seen several patients with osteomyelitis of the foot, and scrubbed in to help with their amputations. Folks with diabetes get these infections for a lot of reasons. Diabetes harms your immune system, making it harder for your body to fight back simple infections. It also attacks the nerves, starting with the small nerves out at the far end of your body.

Feet start to tingle, then hurt, and then they go totally numb. This makes you prone to foot injuries, because you stumble, and then you may not notice an injury. If I cut the bottom of my foot, I'd know immediately. But with bad diabetes, a little injury to the toe can go unnoticed until it blows up into a big infection. That's what we call a "diabetic foot." When antibiotics fail—as they often do in cases of diabetic bone infection, because of the already weakened immune system—surgery is the only option.

At St. Vincent's, I had learned how good primary care can prevent these amputations. We would teach our diabetic patients to check their feet every day. When they come into the clinic, we look for foot injuries, then check the reflexes and sensation in the foot to see how the nerves are doing. It's part of the standard of care for diabetes.

"Sheesh," said my resident. "He's already had one amputation." She was looking down at his chart, where the emergency room doctors had written his history. "You'd think this kid would've learned his lesson."

This kid? I thought, and looked down at the chart. Damien was twenty-one.

The other amputations I'd seen had all been in older people. There was an eighty-year-old transferred from a nursing home, and a fifty-five-year-old severely obese woman, and an immigrant in his sixties. All these people had had diabetes for many years, and they were uninsured in Texas. They weren't getting good primary care.

But why would a twenty-one-year-old already be getting his second amputation? Damien had had diabetes since childhood, but even so, it was unusual for the disease to be so devastating at such a young age. "Let's go talk to him," the resident said.

There's a lot of variation in the quality of rooms in our county ER, and this was not a nice one. The worst "rooms" are just ten-by-eight spaces where one moaning person is separated from the next by curtains. This one had actual walls, but no windows, and was very small. The kid was on a gurney, and he didn't turn to look at us when we came in.

The resident sat by the bed. "Damien," she said gently. He turned and looked at her. "I'm Dr. Sklar."

"You the surgeon?"

"I am."

"You going to cut off my foot?"

The resident looked down. This was, of course, the news we had come to deliver. But she wanted it to come more gently. The kid already knew. "Well," she said, "we need to do surgery."

"Oh no, no, no." He tossed his head back and looked at the wall behind him. "Don't you fucking do that," he said. His voice dropped down to a whisper. "Please don't do that."

"I'm going to try," the resident said, "to take as little as possible." She reached down and touched the top of his foot, above where the infection was. "It looks like your bones are infected up to about here," she said, "so I'm going to try to leave the back half of your foot."

"Please," he said.

"I know this is awful."

Damien half rolled over, turning his back to us. "You don't know shit," he whispered.

THERE WERE, I LEARNED, a lot of reasons why a twenty-one-year-old would already be needing his second amputation. Damien was from Chicago. He was diagnosed with diabetes when he was eight years old. Childhood diabetes is relentless: the pancreas gets totally destroyed, so those kids need insulin every day for their entire lives. They need special diets and regular medical checkups, attention from nutritionists and social workers: a whole, organized, medical team. The family also has to organize itself around taking care of these kids, or else they get bad complications, from infections to coma to early-onset heart disease. Even in the best situations, bad things happen. A friend of mine from a wealthy family, who was a doctor himself, had chronic blackouts from central nervous system complications from his childhood diabetes.

Damien's family couldn't organize itself around caring for him. His dad had been in jail Damien's whole life, and he and his mother and sisters were chronically homeless. He dropped out of school, and had been arrested three times by his eighteenth birthday. He'd ended up in Texas just three months before, coming down to live with a friend. But when the friend lost his apartment, Damien was on the streets again—without insulin. This was not the kind of life that lends itself to the diligent care required to manage diabetes.

Even if Damien had had great access to medical care, there is reason to think that he might not have received the best care. In 2003, partly in response to studies from the 1990s showing that black and Latino patients were less likely to be given adequate analgesia—pain medication—in emergency rooms, the Institute of Medicine (IOM) undertook a major review of racial bias in medical care.* What they found was disturbing: not only was racial bias prevalent across medicine but bias by physicians contributed independently to the earlier deaths of African American men. The studies that the IOM report considered controlled for factors such as socioeconomic status and access to care, and showed that race alone often affects the quality of care patients receive. For example, National Institutes of Health (NIH) researchers found that black veterans treated for their diabetes at Veterans Affairs hospitals were less likely than white veterans to get basic standard-of-care tests like an eye exam—which is particularly important because diabetes can cause blindness. Discouragingly, another 2014 study found that even in a patient-centered medical home run out of an academic medical center in Washington state—which should offer topflight primary care—black diabetes patients got worse care. Doctors were less likely to do eye exams on their black patients, less likely to vaccinate black patients for the flu, and even less likely to check their hemoglobin A1c (a standard test that tells us how the blood sugar has been running on average for the past

---

* Institute of Medicine, "Unequal Treatment: Confronting Racial and Ethnic Disparities in Health Care" (Washington, DC: National Academies Press, 2010), accessed April 10, 2014, http://www.nap.edu/catalog/10260.html.

three months). Black patients in the study population also had higher average blood sugars than whites—placing them at an increased risk for complications like the infection Damien had. The research on this topic goes on and on.

John Dovidio, a sociologist who studies race in medicine, argues that many physicians exhibit "aversive racism." He means that we value equality and condemn the notion that we might be racist, but we still act on subtle, unacknowledged bias. Patients pick up on aversive racism through cues, such as shifty eye movements or the physician leaving the room quickly. And leaving the room quickly is a problem: the shorter doctor visits that patients of color receive may explain why doctors are less likely to hit the standard of care for these patients. Researchers have also examined factors among physicians that contribute to bias, and the results are incomplete, but interesting: physician-patient teams of the same race are less likely to be influenced by bias. This is one reason why it's vitally important to educate a diverse population of doctors.

To evaluate whether physicians have unconscious biases, researchers use a tool called the Implicit Association Test (IAT). This test is available online, and anyone can take it. I did myself, and I got the most troubling possible score: my answers showed that I have a *strong* automatic preference for European Americans as opposed to African Americans. About 27 percent of people in general had gotten this result at the time I took the study, and 27 percent more showed "moderate" preference for European Americans as opposed to African Americans. Sixteen percent had a slight automatic preference, 17 percent showed no preference, and the other 12 percent had slight to strong automatic preference for African Americans. Most white respondents preferred whites, and so did about 50 percent of African American respondents.

My result was, obviously, disturbing. I'd like to think that I'm not that shifty-eyed doctor who rushes out of the room. I trained in an African American community center, have an excellent African American academic mentor, and I've thought about these problems a lot—surely I shouldn't be that biased!

I repeated the test, and got the same result.

This was discouraging. If I'm so biased, could I ever be a good provider for nonwhite patients? Maybe I should just stop trying. My presence in a medical encounter with an African American patient could actually be harmful.

Fleeing from these problems, of course, is not really an option for physicians—and, given how few African American and Latino physicians the medical system trains, it would be disastrous for patients. White docs cannot responsibly wait for a revolution in medical education so that our colleagues of color can "fix" this problem; nor should this issue be the sole purview of physicians of color. We all have to take good care of our patients now. So researchers have come up with some ways that physicians can begin to address bias in our practices.

The IAT originators write that people who show moderate to strong preference for one racial group can avoid letting this influence our behaviors, but only if we make a constant effort. If we stop trying, then bias probably gets back to work. Dovidio and his colleagues argue that there are things we health care providers in particular can do to address implicit bias. This is good news for me, as well as for patients.

The exercises they suggest are pretty simple, and designed to address the factors that make docs more likely to act on bias: stress, anxiety, unfamiliarity, and lack of empathy. For example, to reduce anxiety and unfamiliarity, physicians should talk with colleagues of other races. We should use mindfulness techniques, like meditation, to reduce our anxiety before clinical encounters. We should get to know our patients well, so that we think of them not in terms of categories like race or gender, but in terms of their individual selves. And we should actively empathize by trying to imagine what it would be like to be in our patients' situations. Empathy is a particular sticking point. Because research shows that physician empathy declines throughout our training, any measures we take to foster empathy will probably have to be repeated . . . like, forever.

In much of his writing, Dovidio argues that doctors can begin to address this problem by thinking of ourselves not as a separate group from patients (or members of racial minorities), but rather as members of one overarching group. Humans, say. We could try to remember that we're all human, and we're supposed to be working together.

I ENDED UP TALKING with Damien a lot. I guess it was because I felt guilty for being part of the team that was operating on his foot. Maybe I was just trying to comfort myself, but I thought he might feel better if he had someone to talk to. So I'd drop into his room after rounds, and we'd talk. I don't think it actually made much of a difference to him. In the end, he lost the foot, and that was what he cared about—not connecting with some random, guilty-feeling medical student. When I tried to talk with him about learning to walk again and everything he could still do, he shut me down: "I ain't going to have no kind of life," he said, "with half a foot."

He did tell me a lot about himself, though. He told me how much he loved his mother and how hard she fought for him, hauling him into clinics month after month and getting his paperwork in so he held on to medical coverage, even when they were homeless. He blamed his illness on himself, on running away and getting in trouble, on doing bad things. Teenagers, I told him, always screw up on their diabetic care. When you're that age, it's impossible to know how bad the complications will be. Damien was angry, but mostly at himself.

Things become so immediate in medicine. I was an MD/PhD student, and I could easily find myself zooming out into thoughts about the research on race and bias, and everything that we as a profession could do to change things. But when you're actually doing medicine, you always return to the particular body; every afternoon, I returned to Damien's room. You can say that the medical system has problems, but then there is the actual pus oozing out of the bottom of this particular wound. And this particular young man, whom I found myself caring about, was actually losing his foot.

We did the surgery late that first night. I brought my size-six non-latex surgical gloves to the scrub tech, then washed my hands and scrubbed under my nails. I got to the operating room before the rest of the team, and talked with Damien while the anesthesiologists put him under. There was a black line marked on his foot where we were going to cut. "This drug is for pain. This one's going to make you sleepy. Are you ready? Okay, count backward from ten . . ."

Once he was asleep, we swung into action. We painted his foot with dark-red Betadine and got the overhead lights shining right on it. The senior resident began to cut, while the attending physician observed and I ran a little tube sucking up blood and stray bits of bone. It went quickly. The sick bone crumbled, and we cut away infected tissue until all we could see was healthy looking. We managed to leave his two smallest toes and most of the foot, rinsing the wound thoroughly with sterile water. We bandaged it up, and that was that.

THE NEXT DAY, Damien was playing the snake game on his beat-up mobile phone. We talked a little bit. His pain was okay. He was eating and going to the bathroom. He'd even managed to hobble around a little bit on his crutches.

It was on the third day that he spiked a fever. And when we unwrapped the bandages, the infection was back—despite the antibiotics we were giving him. Thick pus oozed between the exposed bones of his middle foot. The next operation would have to be a BKA—a below-the-knee amputation.

We cut off his whole foot, just above the ankle.

Damien left the hospital a week later. He had prescriptions for insulin and follow-up appointments with our medical team, the surgeon, and a physical therapist. He knew how to clean and check his wound. He'd been signed up for the Medical Assistance Program, so he was going to get his supplies and appointments free or cheaply. When he was healed, he'd be able to get a prosthesis. We did all we could—everything that humane medicine can do in the aftermath of a disaster—but of course he was still angry.

Also, there was nowhere to send him. The friend was still home-less, and Damien didn't want to see him. He couldn't bear to call his mother yet. We sent him out in a taxi, with his crutches, for a three-night guaranteed stay at the Salvation Army.

CHAPTER 14

MY NEXT ROTATION WAS A MONTH OF RURAL FAMILY MED-
icine in Alpine, Texas. Alpine is in the West Texas desert near Big
Bend National Park. It's a gorgeous part of the country and, best of all,
my good friend Margaret was assigned to the same rotation. We made
the six-hour drive from Austin to Alpine in my trusty Honda, Box, and
moved into the house we'd been assigned to by the hospital district.

Margaret and I were grateful for the free digs, but the house was
weird. It was, to my eyes, a mansion. It was owned by a guy who
travels a lot for work, and who apparently shares custody of his son
and daughter. I unpacked in the son's room, where the linens were
all camo themed and a pointillist picture of an eight-year-old holding a crossbow graced the eastern wall. Margaret took the daughter's room, which was flush with giant stuffed unicorns. There was a
Spanish-speaking woman named Marta who cleaned the house and
would make our beds each morning; it made me so uncomfortable
that, for the first time in my life, I started making my bed. In addition
to us and Marta, the house was also shared by a man who worked
for some government agency. He would come home from work with
a gun strapped to his hip, stroll out to the pool—which, y'all, had
fountains that shot from little lions' heads—and try to strike up a
conversation with Margaret. Margaret diligently ignored him.

Margaret and I split our time between the two family doctors in town, Dr. Billings and Dr. Leucke. I started working with Dr. Leucke, who had offices in Alpine and the nearby town of Fort Davis. So on Monday morning, I met Dr. Leucke at the hospital in Alpine. "Hello, hello," he said when I found him. "Rachel, right?" He was a fit middle-aged man with a young-looking face and sandy blond hair. He wore scrub bottoms and a black T-shirt.

"That's me," I said.

"And you're a third-year student?"

"Yes."

"So what have you done so far?"

"Surgery," I said.

"That's it?" he asked.

"That's it."

"Okay, well," he said, "this will be a little bit different."

"Great," I said.

And so it was. We rounded on three patients in the hospital that morning, all of whom Dr. Leucke knew very well. He would say, "Well Roy, how's your breathing?" or "Sandy, have you pooped yet?" then do a brief physical exam, kiss his patient on the head, and scrawl an illegible three-sentence note on the chart. It took about an hour. Then we retired to the hospital cafeteria for breakfast—grits and eggs—before driving out to Fort Davis in Dr. Leucke's SUV. We wound through the Davis Mountains, and each turn showed another beautiful vista: high desert, with the long brown and green landscape stretching out beneath.

"Here's where the Rock House fire was," he said, as we approached Fort Davis. "This was all green. Terrible thing. Affected a lot of the ranchers. One of my patients lost his whole herd, had to start over from nothing."

"That's awful," I said.

"Well, thank god for the public radio station," he said. "They warned everybody in time to get out safe."

On the rest of the drive, I got a little bit of Dr. Leucke's story. He had initially trained as a surgeon, but switched to family medicine. He had two daughters, but his ex-wife had left Alpine after a few years and lived in Abilene now. His daughter called while we were on the road, but the phone dropped the call as we passed behind a ridge. We got cell service again near town, and Dr. Leucke's screen blinked with missed calls—his daughter, and two from patients. All his patients had his cell phone number.

We pulled into Fort Davis, a little strip of a town with one thousand inhabitants, nestled at the foot of the mountains near the McDonald Observatory. The clinic is in a stone building at one end of town, and we walked right in through the waiting room. Dr. Leucke said hi to everybody, then sent me off to see the first patient. "Ooh, it's Mr. Hausen," he said. "Talk him down for me, Rachel. Talk him down."

Mr. Hausen was a rancher in his sixties with sun-weathered skin and strong arms. "I think I tore myself," he said, "picking up a hay bale."

His wife nodded significantly. "Yes he did," she said. *"Down there."*

"I understand," I said. This was bread and butter for me: on my surgery rotation, I had helped repair a bunch of hernias and learned to do a good hernia exam in clinic. Mr. Hausen told me the whole story: how he'd picked up the hay bale and felt a sudden pain in his groin area, and the pain didn't go away.

"Go ahead and pull your jeans down," I said after a while, "and I'll check you for a hernia." Mr. Hausen shrugged his shoulders, said, "Well, all right," and unbuckled his belt. Sure enough, when I pressed my finger up against the opening of his inguinal canal and had him cough, a bulge nudged down against my fingertip.

"Yup," I said. "That's a hernia."

"Well, hell," he said, looking down at his genitals.

"Yup," I repeated. I stood up and took my gloves off.

"Well, hell!" Mrs. Hausen said, pointing at Mr. Hausen's genitals. "It's broken!"

"Yes ma'am," I said. "But, um, it's not too broken. I mean, we can fix it."

"Damn it to hell," Mr. Hausen said, putting his hands on his hips. "I sure as hell hope y'all can fix it."

"That's right," Mrs. Hausen said, nodding vigorously.

"You can go ahead and pull your shorts up," I said. "We'll have Dr. Leucke take a look."

I stepped out, and found Dr. Leucke in the office. "How's Mr. Hausen?" he asked.

"He has a hernia!" I said. "He got it from picking up a hay bale."

"My goodness," Dr. Leucke said.

"It's a left-sided indirect inguinal hernia," I said.

"You checked him for it?"

"I sure did. I did a lot of hernia exams on my surgery rotation," I said.

"Well, well. Good for you," Dr. Leucke said, blushing a little bit.

Back in the exam room, Dr. Leucke had Mr. Hausen pull his jeans down again.

"Yup," Dr. Leucke said. "That's a hernia."

"Well, hell," Mr. Hausen said.

Dr. Leucke turned to me. "You sure did learn how to do a hernia exam!" he said.

"Yes, sir," I said. "Thank you."

"She did a real good job," Mr. Hausen said.

"Yes sir," Mrs. Hausen said. "She sure did."

"Well, thank-y'all," I said.

"Oh, you can pull your jeans up now," Dr. Leucke said. "I reckon we're gonna schedule you for some surgery."

"Up in Alpine?" Mr. Hausen asked.

"Up in Alpine," Dr. Leucke said.

"Well, hell," said Mrs. Hausen. Then she pointed to Mr. Hausen's genitals. "Will it still work?" she asked.

"Yes, ma'am," Dr. Leucke said. "Don't let him fool you. It'll work."

"All right then," she said. Then Dr. Leucke kissed them both on the top of the head and we stepped out.

We saw six more patients before the lunch hour, then Dr. Leucke dismissed me so that he could eat and take a nap on the picnic table behind the clinic. His head nurse had built him a garden back there, and he always liked to nap in the midafternoon. So I wandered over to the drugstore for a sandwich, then took my own nap on the court-house lawn. I took off my white coat and laid on my back on the sunny lawn, watching the buzzards fly slow loops high above the desert.

MY SECOND NIGHT IN ALPINE, I bedded down in the little boy's camouflage bedroom and went to sleep. Around four a.m., my phone rang.

"Hello?" I groaned.

"Hi, Rachel," Dr. Leucke said. "It's Dr. Leucke."

"Hi, Dr. Leucke," I said.

"I reckon you oughta come on down here to the hospital," he said. "We've got a lady in labor, and I think she's about to pop."

Suddenly, I was completely awake. "I'll be right there," I said. I threw off the covers, hauled on my scrubs, and jumped into Box to drive across town.

The moon was high over the desert and the town was asleep. I sped toward the hospital, my heart beating fast. I had never seen a baby born before.

As I approached the outskirts of Alpine, however, red and blue lights flashed in my rearview mirror. I was being pulled over. I pulled to the edge of the road and slumped forward in my seat. I was sure I would miss the delivery. The cop sat behind me, lights flashing. I couldn't stand it. My first baby would be born without me.

Then, I had the bright idea of grabbing my stethoscope off the rearview mirror and sticking it out the window. The cop saw it, and pulled up next to me. He was a young guy.

"Are you going to the hospital?" he asked.

"Yes," I said. "There's a baby being born, and I need to get there right away." For the record, I did not say, *I'm a third-year medical stu-*

dent, and this baby will be delivered with or without me. You could arrest me right now, and it would make zero difference to the mother or the baby.

"Okay, follow me," the cop said. Then he led me through town with his lights flashing, straight to the hospital. Dr. Leucke's truck was parked next to the emergency room doors. I parked next to him, punched in the EMS code, and ran straight in.

THE DELIVERY ROOM was perfectly quiet except for the heavy breathing of the woman in labor. She was alone in there—no husband, no mother, no sisters helping her out. She was flat on her back on the hospital bed, with her legs spread apart in stirrups. Dr. Leucke was at the foot of the bed in a gown and scrub booties, and a nurse was standing next to a tray covered in sterile blue cloth. Another nurse stepped in as I did, and began speaking quietly to the woman in Spanish. "You're doing good, mama," she said. "Keep breathing. You're going good."

"*No puedo!*" the woman gasped.

"Yes, you can," the nurse said. "Yes, you can."

Dr. Leucke turned to me. "You made it!" he said.

"Yes sir," I said. The nurse helped me into a gown and sterile gloves, and I stood next to Dr. Leucke.

"Go ahead and check her," he told me.

I knew what Dr. Leucke meant: I was supposed to check her cervix, to see how far along she was in labor. But this was my first delivery, and I wouldn't really know how to check the cervix, or what I was feeling. I knew, too, that unnecessary vaginal exams during labor can increase the chances of infection for mother and baby.

"Okay," I said.

I didn't want to say, in front of Dr. Leucke and the nurses and this mother, that I had no idea what I was doing. I easily could have. Dr. Leucke is a gentle man, and he wouldn't have gotten mad at me. In retrospect, the calculus of this—embarrassing myself slightly by asking for help, versus putting a mother and a tiny newborn baby at risk—is obvious. But in that moment, I didn't think it through. I just tried to do what I was told.

I stepped between the woman's legs, and stretched my gloved hand toward her vagina. I was nervous and I moved quickly, barely remembering to introduce myself. "I'm Rachel," I said in Spanish. "I'm a medical student working with Dr. Leucke. I'm going to check you now."

She didn't say anything at all to me.

I pressed my index and middle fingers toward where I thought was the vagina.

"You gonna check her?" Dr. Leucke asked.

"Um, yes sir," I said.

"Well, that's the anus. Better wash your glove," Dr. Leucke said. *You complete idiot,* I told myself. *You just tried to stick your fingers in a woman's anus during labor. You can't even find the vagina when it's about to deliver a baby.* I flushed bright red. Behind me, the nurses were silent. One held out a tray of fluid for me to wash my glove.

Still nervous and moving quickly, I dipped my glove in the fluid, splashed it around a little, and quickly turned back to the woman, feeling almost panicky. This woman was in labor, and I had just violated her body. I felt mortified and awful. I wished that Dr. Leucke would banish me from the delivery room, or that the woman would sit up on her bed and demand that the medical student who clearly had no idea what she was doing be pilloried. But they didn't. I was allowed—asked—to carry on.

This time, at least, I managed to correctly identify the vagina. I moved my hand as gently as I could into her vagina. Inside, I could feel the hard round orb of the baby's head pushing through her cervix.

"Where's she at?" Dr. Leucke said.

"Um," I said, "about eight."

"All right," he said. "All right." I had no idea if I was right. I was guessing she was dilated to eight centimeters, just because I could tell she was pretty close. But actually, I had no idea.

I didn't have time to stop feeling nervous before the woman started pushing. The nurse stood by her head, encouraging her. "Okay, Rachel," Dr. Leucke said. "You just stand here by me, and catch him like a football."

"Like a football?" I asked. We didn't have a football team in Port Aransas.

"Yeah, just catch him with your whole body and cradle him. Babies are slippery. You don't want to drop him."

So that's what I did. The mother gave a loud yell, and suddenly the baby's head popped right out of the mom's vagina. Just the head. It was surreal and for one stunned moment I thought, *Oh my god, that's a human head.*

Then I remembered that of course, of course it was supposed to be there. Dr. Leucke guided the baby's shoulders out, and all at once the boy slithered into my arms, bloody and wet and hot from the inside of his mother's body. He was, for that moment, the most brand new human being in all the world.

"Good job, mama," the nurse said. I was staring down at the baby. He was red and wrinkled and angry, and as soon as Dr. Leucke took him from me, he began to cry.

"Go ahead and clamp that cord," Dr. Leucke said. He showed me where to clamp it. "Usually, we have the dad cut it, but he's not here. She's up from Mexico. You go ahead and cut the cord, Rachel."

So I did. I cut the cord, and then held it taut as the woman's uterus clamped down to deliver the placenta. Finally, with a gush of bright blood, the placenta slithered out. It was purple and it reminded me of a big jellyfish washed up on the beach. *People eat these things*, I thought, looking at it. Then I watched as the baby was weighed, checked over quickly, and handed to his mother. He was absolutely perfect, and she smiled and lay back on her pillow.

We pulled off our bloody smocks, said congratulations to the mother, and headed out. "Go get some sleep, Rachel," Dr. Leucke said. "I'll see you back here at eight."

————

"I DELIVERED MY FIRST BABY LAST NIGHT," I told Margaret over coffee a couple of hours later.

"Was it so, so beautiful?" she asked.

"Sure," I said. "It was beautiful. But I was terrified. And I fucked up trying to check her."

"Mmm, that's okay," Margaret said. "Normal. Did you catch it?"

"Him," I said. "Yeah."

"Nice! How was the delivery?"

"It was pretty old-school," I said. "I think."

"Oh yeah?" Margaret asked.

"Yeah, like, the woman on her back in stirrups instead of walking around or squatting or whatever. We cut the cord immediately, and then the baby was weighed and stuff before he was handed to his mother."

"Old-school for sure," Margaret said.

I finished my coffee and headed back to the hospital to meet Dr. Leucke. I was excited to see the baby, but he was gone. "He had a little cough, maybe a touch of pneumonia," Dr. Leucke explained. "So we sent him out to Odessa."

The mortified flush that I had felt when I messed up the woman's genital exam rushed through me again, only this time it wasn't just about me messing up, or about the woman being violated during labor.

This time, it was about the baby. Pneumonia in a newborn is usually caused by *E. coli*. The *E. coli* could have been introduced by my glove, during the vaginal exam I messed up. I had touched the anus, rushed through washing my glove, and plunged my hand back into the birth canal. I felt sick, like this tiny baby's pneumonia was entirely my fault. I had caused it by trying to do what I was told instead of confessing to the fact that I had no idea what I was doing.

Worst of all, the exam I had done was entirely for practice— it offered no benefit to the mother. And she, being in the middle of labor, being a Spanish-speaking woman delivering in a foreign country—well, she really had no way to refuse.

My very first baby was in an ICU in Odessa, getting antibiotics dripped into his blood and oxygen blown into his face instead of lying in his mother's arms. And it was pretty much my fault.

A few days later, Dr. Leucke let me know that the baby had recovered just fine and was on his way home. I breathed a sigh of relief, but I vowed not to forget my lesson. If I didn't confess to my own ignorance on the wards, I could be putting my patients in danger.

THE NEXT DELIVERY I SAW was an emergency cesarean section. This time, it happened during the day. I was working with the other doc in town, Dr. Billings, at his office near the Alpine hospital. We were in the middle of scraping a suspicious bump of skin off a farmhand's back when a nurse poked her head into the room. "The hospital needs you now, Dr. Billings," she said.

Dr. Billings and I wrapped up the procedure and hopped in his Jeep to go to the hospital. He joked that he could use a flashing light on top, but in the meantime I could roll down my window and make a siren noise. "Cops don't really stop you anymore around here once they know you're the doctor," he explained, "but I like to let people know when it's really an emergency."

That seemed fair enough. Last week, Dr. Leucke had told me a story about driving ninety-five miles an hour from Fort Davis to Alpine for an emergency delivery. The local cops knew him, too, but apparently Dr. Leucke whizzed right past a state trooper who didn't recognize his car. The trooper started chasing him, and by the time they got close to Alpine they had set up a roadblock to stop the doctor. "I made it to the delivery, though," Dr. Leucke said. "That kid is on the football team now."

Dr. Billings and I rushed into the hospital and straight to the operating room. "Have you assisted on a C-section before?" he asked me as we headed in.

"Um, no," I said.

"But you did surgery, so you have some idea what to do?"

"Yes sir," I said.

"Okay, change and meet me in there," he said. "We'll scrub up once she's anesthetized."

The operating room was in the very center of the small hospital. It was so quiet and contained in there that it felt like a church. I changed into a pair of scrubs and found Dr. Billings already in the OR. The nurse anesthetist nodded to me, and I went to meet the patient. She was calm, and young, and sitting up. Her face looked open and trusting, even as the pain of labor washed across it with each long contraction. She pointed to her chest and said her name, "Maria Dolores."

Maria Dolores, I thought. *The suffering of Mary.*

"*Soy* Rachel," I said. "*La estudiante de medicine trabajando con* Dr. Billings" [I'm Rachel, the medical student working with Dr. Billings]. She nodded, and her eyes moved back down to her belly. Dr. Billings gently moved her to the side of the bed, and had her sit up so the anesthetist could put a needle in her back for spinal anesthesia. Spinal anesthesia is similar to an epidural, but it works faster and doesn't last as long, so we often use it rather than epidurals for cesarean sections. You would give an epidural to control pain throughout a labor that could last many hours, whereas a spinal is good for rapid anesthesia in surgery.

The lights in the operating room were all dim, except for one bright light shining down over Maria Dolores. Her legs dangled over the side of the operating table; her feet were small and bare. Dr. Billings stood in front of her to steady her as the nurse anesthetist prepared to put the needle in her spine. He placed his arms around her so that the light fell on his arms and shoulders, and she leaned forward so that the side of her face rested against his chest. All was quiet, and then I could hear Dr. Billings praying over her as the needle slid in.

When Maria Dolores was lying on her back on the operating table, Dr. Billings and I stepped out to scrub. "She's had a C-section before," he explained to me. "And she was going to try to deliver vaginally, but the baby's heart monitor started showing sudden, extreme decelerations. So we're doing this stat. We're going to cut right down her belly instead of across. You'll see the difference when you do your ob-gyn rotation. A scheduled C-section uses a low transverse cut. This is a stat. It's different."

Back in the operating room, the moment of quiet before the surgery was over. We stepped in and began moving very quickly. The nurses had poured Betadine all over Maria Dolores's belly, and Dr. Billings made a long cut and then we both put our hands in the edges of the cut to tear it wider. Blood spilled out the edges of the cut, over the side of the operating table and onto the floor.

"Look at that, look at that, Rachel," Dr. Billings said when we were inside. Instead of the thick muscular wall of the uterus that I expected to see underneath the skin of her belly, there was only a thin membrane. I could see the hair of the baby's head just underneath.

"She already perfed," Dr. Billings said. That is, Maria Dolores's uterus had broken open from the force of her contractions, probably along the line where her uterus had been cut before. "If this had taken five minutes longer," he said, and didn't finish. The tissue-thin amniotic membrane was the only thing keeping this baby from floating free in her mother's abdomen.

Dr. Billings carefully opened the amniotic membrane and began to maneuver the baby out. "It's a girl!" he said. "She's breathing!" And as soon as he had said it, miraculously, the baby girl began to cry. A minute later, I was crying, too. Some things in medicine really are miraculous; there's no other word.

THE NEXT SATURDAY I was back with Dr. Leucke for his monthly trip out to the free clinic in Candelaria. This clinic is funded entirely by donations from the Lutheran church, in which Dr. Leucke is an elder. It doesn't take much once the doctor volunteers his time—a few hundred dollars a month for basic antibiotics and other medicines, supplies, and the cost of lab tests. Plus toys for the local kids. Dr. Leucke transports the clinic supplies in big Tupperware boxes in the back of his SUV.

Candelaria is a *colonia*—one of the border towns so poor and so isolated that they don't even have city services. We drove through the desert for an hour and a half, first through the mountain pass and then through Presidio, the American town across the river from Ojinaga. Ojinaga has somewhere between twenty thousand and seventy thousand inhabitants—nobody seems to know for sure. But there's a hospital there. In Presidio, there are only clinics. Presidio also has a dusty grocery store, a lot of rusting cars, and the shotgun shacks surrounded by barbed wire where the Border Patrol workers live. They look like the FEMA houses in Galveston, and may have been built by the same people.

After Presidio, we turned north to follow the path of the river toward Candelaria. The road was paved until we got within a few miles, and then it became a dirt track. Candelaria was just a cluster of houses along a few dirt roads beside the river. "The kids here take the school bus into Presidio," Dr. Leucke said. "It's two and a half hours on the bus every day. You want groceries, you want batteries, you want a pair of socks . . . Presidio."

Kids ran up to the SUV when Dr. Leucke pulled up next to a small adobe church. He hopped out and started saying hello to them and handing around toys—mostly bright, bouncy balls. "I delivered half these kids," he told me. The kids scattered and began chasing one another around in the sunshine, scattering up dust.

We walked into the church, which was cool and dim. People were waiting for us in there—three or four moms with little kids, an elderly couple, and a few younger people on their own. "*Hola,* doctor," a woman called out. Dr. Leucke said hello, introduced me, and we set to work.

We set up the clinic inside the church itself, in a chapel that had been converted into an exam room thanks to a donated bed. Christ on the cross watched everything we did—*a particularly gory Christ,* I thought, with blood painted down the sides of his face. Dr. Leucke set up for a while on one end of the church's nave so that I could do pap smears on the exam bed in the chapel. They all went smoothly. I put the samples in a little cooler to be taken back to Alpine for analysis, and let the women know that we would have their results next month. I felt bad for them—waiting on pap smear results is stressful. It would be hard to wait a whole month.

In this incredibly resource-poor setting, we practiced in a different way. Kids who had viral illnesses would sometimes get antibiotics. Dr. Leucke would have me explain to their moms in Spanish: "Don't give him the antibiotics yet. You only need them if he isn't getting better by Wednesday. If he still has fever, or he's getting worse, then he can start taking the antibiotics." The pills were meant to cover for the possibility of a bacterial infection developing. Next week, the nearest doctor would be in Presidio, and he'd only be there Tuesday and Thursday. So, if a kid started to go downhill, Dr. Leucke wanted them to have antibiotics on hand already. We would also give the moms bottles of ibuprofen for fever, and sometimes cough syrup.

Patients kept coming all afternoon. Half were from Candelaria, and half had waded across the river from the little Mexican town there. Everyone spoke Spanish, and only the junior high and high school–age kids spoke English. It wasn't just viral illnesses, either—one kid was a cancer survivor, one woman had a rare lung disease that Dr. Leucke had caught, and some of the elderly people were pretty frail.

Late in the afternoon, we ran out of antibiotics. There was just one more family to see—a mother and two kids who had come over to the clinic from Mexico. The mom explained that her kids were sick—feverish and shaking, with sore throats.

"Okay, let's have a look," Dr. Leucke said. And sure enough, both the two-year-old and the five-year-old looked bad. You know a two-year-old is sick when he doesn't even try to fight you putting your otoscope in his ear. His ears were clear, but I saw white patches all over his tonsils. He was feverish at 102 degrees, and I also felt small, hard, swollen lymph nodes down the sides of his neck.

"I think he has strep throat," I told Dr. Leucke. Dr. Leucke nodded. The five-year-old had it, too.

"I wish we still had some amoxicillin," Dr. Leucke said. "These
kids are really sick."

Strep throat is not exactly a medical emergency, but it has to be
treated. In the days before penicillin was widely available, strep throat
killed a lot of people. If left untreated, it can lead to rheumatic fever,
and rheumatic heart disease, and early death. The use of penicillin
and related antibiotics to treat strep infections is one of the simple,
cheap cures of which medicine should be most proud. But at this
moment, in this improvised clinic in an adobe church on the Mexico
border, we were out of amoxicillin.

I expected Dr. Leucke to do something bold at this moment—to
load the kids in his car to take them to Presidio, or to tell the mom
she needed to get them to Ojinaga urgently for antibiotics. But he
didn't. He comforted the mother, gave her Tylenol to keep the kids'
fevers down, and sent them on their way. He let her know that it was
a bacterial infection, but we were out of antibiotics. If she could make
the trip to Ojinaga, she should. She nodded and thanked us, but her
brow was furrowed with worry.

We broke down the clinic and loaded it back into the SUV after
they left, then we drove home slowly on the unpaved mountain road,
past the Chinati Hot Springs. The sun set over Big Bend, bathing the
mountains in pink and orange. Dr. Leucke and I were quiet.

"I wish we hadn't run out of antibiotics," he finally said. "Those
last two were really sick."

Back at the mansion that night, I thought of those two kids shivering and sweating in their house across the river. I looked up the
incidence of rheumatic fever in kids with untreated strep throat. How
many would get that condition, which would limit and likely shorten
their lives? The answer was 3–5 percent. But would those kids get it?
Would they make it to Ojinaga? I'd never know.

Dr. Leucke's little free clinic on the border was miraculously cheap, and it was okay medicine: we caught some things, treated some things, did some screening tests. But it was not the best medicine, and I felt that these people, who were so poor, really needed the best. What if the presence of the monthly free clinic kept them from going into Presidio or Ojinaga, where they could get better care?

I had heard similar arguments made about St. Vincent's: some people think free clinics are altogether a bad idea, that we are a stop-gap measure designed to help medical professionals feel better about injustice in medicine. My friend Merle called St. Vincent's "a moral safety valve"—the fact that it existed allowed UTMB employees to keep practicing in an unjust system without our anger or frustration boiling over, because it made us feel like we were doing some good even inside a broken system. Merle worries that free clinics don't really help the community as much as they help students (who need the training) and providers (who need to feel like we are moral people, donating our expertise for charity).

In Galveston, though, there was always the counterargument: There was no other option for most of our patients. Even with the help of St. Vincent's, some would die of treatable diseases. It would be cruel to abandon them completely, when I had no real faith that the system would step in to pick up the slack.

I tossed and turned in bed that night, thinking these questions over. Was second-rate care better than no care at all? What would it feel like to place your life in the hands of students, or of charity? I thought of the laboring mother from Mexico who had birthed her boy here, in the country with the most technologically sophisticated medical system in the world, only to have him sent to Odessa with pneumonia because of a medical student's nervous stupidity. She was probably sitting by his crib now, in a dark NICU room shepherded by machines, listening to each fragile breath. I wished I could sit with her a while, so that I, too, could reassure myself that the boy was still breathing. So that I could say I was sorry.

Then I thought of the other mother, who had waited on the pew of an adobe church with two boys shivering from fever. We had let her cross the river again with only Tylenol to treat them. Any of those boys could die—soon, or later.

I thought of Dr. Leucke kissing his patients on the head, giving out his cell phone number, living across the state from his family. I was, frankly, afraid to become like these Alpine doctors, who had given up so much to practice family medicine. *He loves his patients*, I thought, *but is it possible to do right by them this way*? The dark lay thick over the desert all around me, and I lay awake for a long time.

CHAPTER 15

THE PROBLEMS OF RURAL MEDICINE FELT PERSONAL TO ME, not only because of my upbringing and my training in Alpine but also because of my brother, Matt.

Matt grew up to be a fisherman, as we all knew he would. He started deckhanding in Port Aransas at fourteen years old, and moved to Alaska when he finished his undergraduate philosophy degree. His first job there was on a cod-fishing boat in the Bering Sea. He would stand on the deck and gaff cod after cod as they rose shining and struggling from the water, hooked by the long-liner, before they were pulled into a machine called the crucifier and then shuttled down into the freezing hold. On one trip, so much ice fog froze in the high rigging of the ship that it threatened to capsize them, and the whole crew had to spend three days with picks and jackhammers breaking ice. Capsizing meant death, and that's the way most people die in the Bering Sea—all together, when the ship goes down. The work can tear your body down, rip your digits off, or lame you, but death is generally a group affair.

Matt tells a story of a crew that got caught in the cabin of a capsizing boat because they put on their survival suits—bright orange jumpsuits that float and keep you warm—in the cabin, and couldn't get out when the vessel immersed. He tells another story of a crew that died from the poison fumes in a cabin when the boat flipped over, burning. Whole crews of thirty that just disappeared in the waves and fog. I would wait for Matt's monthly phone calls while I worked summer internships in my latter years in Austin, trying not to think about those stories.

Nowadays, Matt runs a salmon troller that docks in Craig, Alaska. Craig is a thirty-minute floatplane ride from Ketchikan on Prince of Wales Island. The area is basically a flooded mountain range, where towering firs grow right down to the edge of the water. Seen from above, Craig is small and bright on the island, home to fourteen hundred Alaskans and more tourists in the summer, plus plenty of bears and eagles. Like West Texas, Alaska feels freer because it is wild. One of the freedoms you might have in this part of the world is to start a fish-processing plant on a semiremote island, and then call the town that springs up around it after your first name: Craig.

If you go out to visit Matt, he'll just wait on his boat until he sees the floatplane go over, then walk down to the dock to be there, grinning through his wild beard, as your plane touches down gently by the harbor. Matt's boat, the *Viking Rover*, is a small operation that he can actually run entirely by himself. The *Viking Rover* is a troller, not a trawler. (A troller is a small boat that catches fish on lines, often by hand; a trawler is a larger operation that uses nets.) Matt's boat is also his home. It is stocked not only with gaffs and lures and survival suits but also with fast-cooking Irish oatmeal, tobacco, a shotgun, a pair of gray fleece slippers, and piles of books. The last time I went to visit Matt, he was reading a book about the colonization of British North America. In his bunk, there was a Dave Eggers novel, Anne Applebaum's *Gulag*, and a book by William Barrett called *Irrational Man: A Study in Existential Philosophy*. Matt would anchor nights in a pretty cove near a bed of kelp where sea otters like to nap, and sit up a while after twelve hours of hard fishing, reading about the clash of civilizations and spitting tobacco overboard out the window. The *Viking Rover* is, in my opinion, damn cozy.

Matt sleeps lightly when the boat is anchored. He's attuned to boat noises, and the littlest sound can wake him: a rope rubbing, a change in the wind direction, even the sudden silence of a lull. He'll go out after the salmon for five days at a time, so he spends most nights during the fishing season anchored in some cove near wherever he's fishing. The *Viking Rover* has an anchor alarm that sounds a soft beep if the anchor starts dragging across the seabed—as it might do if the wind kicks up at three a.m.—and Matt will spring up out of his bunk at the beep, throw on a pair of shorts, and hustle out onto the deck to haul up and reposition the anchor while the *Viking Rover* rolls and bucks. If Matt didn't wake up, he'd risk losing the boat if she ran into rocks or into another boat anchored nearby.

He gets up for good around five a.m., hauls up the anchor, turns on the radio, and motors out to start trolling. The cabin is heated by a diesel stove, so Matt nudges the kettle over onto the hottest part of the stovetop to heat water for his morning coffee. When he gets close to a fishing spot, he puts the boat on autopilot and goes out to the aft deck—the back of the boat, also called the cockpit—to set the fishing gear.

The *Viking Rover* is a power troller. It's a thirty-six-foot boat with a central mast and two high outriggers, which are poles that form a *V*-shape on either side of the mast when not in use. When engaged, the outriggers drop down parallel to the boat to hold the gear out from the sides of the boat, so that four long cable lines can run down toward the bottom at once. Each cable has a heavy steel sinker at the bottom, about the size of a honeydew melon. These sinkers sit in holders on the back of the boat when the gear is up. To set the gear, you lift up a sinker out of its holder so that it dangles over the side. Then, you engage the power winch so the sinker slowly trundles down. There are spacers set about every ten feet all along the cable, and as the sinker goes down you clip a leader onto each spacer. The leaders are basically heavy strands of fishing line with lures tied to the end. So Matt clips around fifteen lures to a cable as it trundles down, flipping his arm back to make sure the hooks dangle free out into the water, then sets the brake on the winch and moves to the next cable. Once all four cables are set, he heads back into the cabin for coffee and the boat moves slowly along, dragging the lures. There are springs on the outriggers that bounce and tighten when a fish comes on, so Matt has some idea of how the catch is going.

Matt'll troll along for anywhere from twenty minutes to an hour, depending on what kind of action he sees in the springs. When it's time to haul gear, he heads back to the cockpit again and engages the winch in reverse to start hauling up a cable. Back there in the cockpit, he can see the bright flashes of free lures or the shine of a salmon as the hooks come up. When there's a fish on, he stops the winch and grabs a gaff. He pulls the fish up close to the boat with one gloved hand, and then smacks it quickly over the head with the club end of the gaff. This stuns or kills the fish. Then he gaffs it through the head and hauls it up onto the boat, where he slits the gill rakers with a small knife so the fish bleeds out. Matt explains that this is a quick way for the fish to die: instead of asphyxiating in the air and suffering, they die fast. Matt cares about fish more than anyone I've ever known—he thinks they're neat animals, and beautiful, and he loves them—so I trust him on this point.

I like helping out on the boat, but the one thing I can't do is club the fish. The first time I tried, it took me three swings to hit the right spot. "That's what you're looking for," Matt said. "That little shudder that means they're dying." But my poor fish had been hit about the shoulders twice before it shuddered, and dangled around in the air while I struggled to get it into position at the side of the boat. I tried again on the next fish, but that time I held the gaff too loosely and it went flying behind me toward the center of the boat.

"Whoa," Matt said, as the gaff whizzed past him.

"I don't think I want to slug the fish," I said.

"Okay, no problem," Matt said. "But you know, it is a really decent way for them to go, all things considered."

"I don't mind that they get clubbed," I said. "I'd just rather they get clubbed once by somebody who will do it right the first time, instead of getting knocked around and hurt by me."

"Right on," Matt said. "I understand."

The truth is, I had had enough of that kind of thing—hurting other living beings in my process of learning—in medical school. Since I wasn't going to be a career deckhand, there was no point in my hurting any fish so that I could learn to do it right. So after that, I stuck to setting gear, manning the wheel to avoid logs and big bunches of kelp while Matt was in the cockpit, and cleaning fish.

I clean fish like a true medical student: carefully, precisely, and slow as hell. The cleaning matters a lot on a salmon boat, because the fish get graded number 1 or number 2 back at port, and number 2s—which have damage to the muscular fillets on the side of the fish, or leftover gore around the head—are worth less money. Matt says that a fast fish cleaner can do two salmon in a minute, ripping out gills, guts, and blood vessels, and tossing them to the gulls behind the boat. I probably average about one salmon every four minutes. I get distracted by the anatomy, wondering why this salmon has such a big liver or puzzling over markings on the scales. I notice the wounds that the salmon have survived: big gashes to the belly or the side, where their intestines have adhered to the sidewall just like human intestines do after a wound. Some fish have lost whole fins, and I ran my hands over the atrophied muscles that must've moved that fin. *It's just like in people*, I thought: When a nerve is cut or a limb is lost, the corresponding muscles waste away. And just like humans, the salmon were able to survive and heal from some pretty massive injuries. It was humbling to me as a medical student to be reminded how capable the body is of healing itself—even in salmon, which obviously have no access to medical care.

Once I get the haul cleaned, I pack them in ice down in the hold of the boat, or in big ice-slush totes on deck.

One reason Matt likes the salmon trolling is that there's practically zero by-kill. Any fish that we can't keep, Matt releases from the hook. Sometimes the lowest hooks will pull up bright-orange rockfish, which are doomed by the sudden change in pressure as they are hauled to the surface. Their eyes bulge and their air bladders swell so that they can't swim back down. As Matt pulls them off the hook and tosses them out, he says, "Eagle's gonna get lucky." And sure enough, a big bird will swoop down to carry away the poor rockfish, which no doubt regrets ever eating that shiny lure.

When a salmon shakes out the hook at the last minute, Matt shrugs and says, "Fish wins." When one salmon shook the hook out so hard that it flew back and embedded in Matt's rain gear, he said, "I'm hooked." Then, after a pause, he added, "This was probably the most resounding fish win of the day."

Matt truly wants to wake up every day and kill two hundred salmon, but he also respects the fish. He has little patience for the environmentalists who only care about mammals—*What about fish? Fish are so important and so neat. Nobody cares about fish just because they don't have cute furry faces*—or who want to preserve wilderness completely free of human access. People need to get to wilderness, he believes, and you shouldn't have to be rich enough to hire an eco tour to be able to use it. Matt cares about conservation that will keep wilderness wild, but open, and he supports fisheries management that will keep fish populations strong but also allow men and women like him to earn a living trolling. And don't even ask him about farmed salmon. Salmon farms raising Atlantic salmon on the Pacific coast have loosed a whole new, non-native species on the ecosystem Matt loves.

Our friend Margaret tells a story of going fishing for white bass with Matt on the Llano River in Texas. They fished all day, and they caught quite a few, but Matt found excuses to let every single fish go. He would pick them up and marvel at them for a minute, then say how this fish was really pretty but probably too small to keep. He'd place it back in the water and watch it swim away. Later in the day, Margaret pulled in a nice-size bass, but Matt said, "This is a nice fish, but really we're not going to catch enough at this point to have a mess." So he gently unhooked the big bass and watched it swim away. You might think it's a paradox for a man who kills fish for a living to love them so much. But if you knew Matt, you'd understand.

———

I ALSO SEE THE *Viking Rover* with the eye of a medical student. The hydraulic-powered winches are relentless, and would rip off a finger if Matt got caught in them. The cables that hang down around the sides of the boats are hazards for tripping and busting open your head. Gaffs and knives and hooks are everywhere. And what about the big diesel engine that rumbles in the belly of the ship, separated from the cabin by just a few planks and a plastic-coated carpet? Matt hauls up these planks to go work on the engine, which is old-timey enough that he can fix it with wrenches instead of having to call in a technician with a computer. But the engine will burn him if he goes in when it's too hot, or could spill fumes into the cabin if something gets misrouted. The larger danger of commercial fishing is obvious: it's the sea itself. But I see all the little things that could maim my brother or even kill him in an accident, especially if he's out on the *Viking Rover* alone. The little things can really get you in isolated places: food poisoning that makes you pass out so the boat rides up on rocks, small cuts that get infected, dehydration.

Matt is attentive to such things. In fact, if you ever want to feel safe in a dangerous place, I recommend being the little sister of a commercial fisherman. My first night on the boat, he oriented me to the fire extinguishers (there are five), showed me my survival suit, told me the difference between smoke flares and parachute flares, and taught me how to use the emergency radio. He also taught me enough about running the boat that I could get out of a tight spot alone if I needed to. Just before I rowed the dinghy out to a nearby kelp bed to look at some otters, Matt told me a story about a guy who died when his dinghy blew past his boat and out into a current. He was pushed out to sea, and eventually drowned. So Matt made me wear a giant, bright red coat with a built-in life jacket and an emergency beacon as I rowed about one hundred yards to look at the otters.

On the boat, I began to realize that the stories these fishermen tell about deaths at sea serve a purpose. I wouldn't put on my survival suit inside the cabin; I would be sure to keep one eye on the *Viking Rover* during my dinghy trip. Those stories could save my life. They reminded me of the stories surgeons tell at their weekly morbidity and mortality conferences, when the whole department reviews the details of cases in which patients died or were hurt. Sometimes, M&M conferences lead surgeons to change some aspect of the system—for example, to move recovery beds closer to the nurses' station, or to increase the number of bags of type O negative blood kept in the emergency room. But even when deaths lead to no such change, talking about mistakes—knowing the story—could prevent another surgeon from making the same error. I wish that more doctors spoke openly about our errors, and that our shame did not prevent us from doing so.

Thinking back over medical school, I could only remember two times outside of M&M when doctors described making mistakes. The first was a lighthearted story from an old neurologist telling how he accidentally hit an artery when trying to draw blood for the first time. He almost fainted when blood went squirting across the room.

The second story was more frightening; indeed, it was intended to frighten us. A surgeon who was leading a small classroom session one day got angry when we second-years couldn't list the criteria for judging liver failure. She was a transplant surgeon, and had a fearsome intellect. "I can't believe you students," she said, stalking back and forth at the front of the classroom. "This is pathetic. If you don't learn your stuff, you're going to kill people." Then she told about a death on the operating table.

A mother was donating her kidney to her young daughter, who had renal failure after a bad infection. Mother and daughter were brought into operating rooms side by side, so the transplant team could move the healthy kidney immediately into the girl's body. The girl was anesthetized and her kidneys were removed. A surgery resident was told to give her a medication so she wouldn't reject her mother's kidney. The resident made a mistake: he pushed the medication, which was a protein, directly into the girl's IV. She went into anaphylactic shock, and died right there on the table.

In the adjacent operating room, the team had already cut the ureter on her mother's kidney.

"That resident should've known," the surgeon said. "It was basic knowledge that you get in these preclinical courses. He should've known, but he didn't, and he killed that little girl. He has to live with that for the rest of his life."

The classroom had grown very quiet.

These are the kinds of error stories you hear as a medical student: the ones that suggest that your stupidity, laziness, or failure to study will make you kill people. They are terrifying and they do serve a purpose. People's lives are in our hands.

I wonder, though, about all the other errors—the ones that don't lead to deaths, but to delays, frustrations, and unnecessary procedures. The small errors—or the ones that can seem small—like forgetting to report the results of a urine sample. Stories about that kind of error need not be designed to terrify us, but rather to help us learn from the mistakes of those who have gone before. After hearing the stories told by these fishermen, I began to realize that I could benefit a lot from hearing more such stories from the doctors training me.

When I think about the mistakes I made at St. Vincent's, I often feel all alone with them. Perhaps talking about them could not only help other students like me feel less ashamed but could prevent them from making the same mistakes that I did. Perhaps, I thought, the medical system could learn something from these fishermen, too.

THERE IS A DOCTOR IN CRAIG, who is good enough that everybody on the dock says they're lucky to have him. "If you get him," a fisherman named John told me, "you know you're in good hands."

One year, he sewed up a nasty, infected cut on my brother's hand. Matt slashed his palm down through fat and muscle to the bone with a fillet knife. He wasn't far from Craig, so he wrapped the hand in a T-shirt and motored into town.

Up at the doctor's office, Matt gaped down at the cut. As used as he is to fish gore, seeing his own body cut open was different. The doctor had splayed open the wound so he and his nurse could clean it out, and Matt looked down to see his white bone glistening through layers of fat and bleeding muscle.

"Wow," Matt said. "That's gross."

"I guess that's pretty gross," the nurse said, pouring pink antiseptic fluid into the wound. "Doctor, should I get the suture kit?"

"Please do," the doctor said. He shot a few injections of lidocaine into the wound along the edges of the skin, and began to sew.

"I've seen a lot grosser," the nurse said.

"I'm sure you have," Matt said. He was feeling a little woozy, watching the needle dip in and out of his hand.

"Wanna hear about the grossest thing I ever saw?" the nurse said.

"Well, sure," Matt said.

"It was a bar fight in Ketchikan. Two loggers. They started out punching each other, but at one point they got in real close and were kind of grappling. Then one logger leaned in and just clean bit the other guy's ear off."

"My, my!" Matt said. "That is gross."

"Oh, that's not the gross part," the nurse said, dabbing blood away from the far edge of Matt's wound as the doctor stitched toward it. "Wanna hear the really gross part?"

"Sure I do," Matt said.

"Well. That one logger had bit off the other logger's ear, and then he just spat it out onto the floor of the bar. When that ear hit the barroom floor, his dog ran right up and ate it. It was like the dog was trained to do it!"

"Wow," Matt said.

"Isn't that gross?"

"Yes, ma'am," Matt said. "That's pretty gross."

When his hand was all sewn up, the doctor explained that Matt had cut into two of the tendons that work his fingers. They were still attached, but it was hard to tell if they would heal on their own or rupture where they'd been cut. "Honestly," the doctor said, "you might want to go out to Anchorage and get an MRI, because you'll be wanting a surgeon to reattach those tendons if they rupture."

"An MRI?" Matt asked. "How expensive is that?"

"It's about five thousand bucks."

"Plus the surgery."

"Yup, plus the surgery. You'd be needing a hand surgeon for this. Might have to go down to the lower forty-eight; I don't think there's a hand surgeon in Alaska right now."

"And what happens if I don't do it?"

"Well, tendons heal pretty slowly because they don't get a lot of blood flow. So we won't know for a few weeks at least if you're out of the woods. If these tendons of yours happen to rupture, you could lose the use of your index finger and your thumb."

Matt was in a tight spot. This was in 2009, and he was uninsured. But he was also a fisherman, and wouldn't be able to do his work without his hands. Even if he could've somehow paid for the MRI and surgery, taking time off work in the middle of the fishing season to get back and forth to Anchorage, and possibly down to Oregon or Washington for surgery, would be a disaster. He'd lose a good chunk of the income that he counts on to pay off his boat and get him through the year. Missed fishing days can't be made up.

There was no way to do it. So he paid the doctor for the stitches and went back to work. He tried to take it easy on his hand for the next few weeks, knowing that another little accident would mean losing his ability to work. The hand stayed sore for a long time, and the fingers never have moved quite like they used to. They get stiff when he works long days. But the tendons didn't rupture, and so Matt can keep on fishing.

CHAPTER 16

AFTER RETURNING TO AUSTIN FROM MY FAMILY MEDICINE rotation, I spent a month on the neurosurgery team. One afternoon that first week on neurosurgery, I squeezed into a room so full of people that I could hardly edge in. At the center, a thin nineteen-year-old boy lay very still on his hospital bed. His mother sat with her hands on his chest, listening to the neurosurgeon.

"I wish I had better news for you," he was saying. "But the CT scan this morning shows what we were afraid of. The cancer is in his brain again."

He paused as a shudder ran through the room. The boy's mother shook her head slowly, lowered her eyes. "We can do surgery, but to get to the lesion we will have to cut through brain tissue. So, just like before, you know the risks. There's a chance of dying in surgery. And afterward, we can't predict what brain damage there might be. You might not be able to move your hands anymore, or understand language. We just don't know."

A stern-faced man spoke up: "And if we don't do the surgery?"

The doctor paused again. "Well, forgoing the surgery in this case would mean that Elias would likely pass away."

"How long?"

"Not long, I think. It's impossible to know for sure, but maybe in a day, maybe a few days. The tumor is bleeding and pressing on his brain, and so he would likely lose consciousness fairly soon. The choice is up to Elias." The doctor's voice lowered. "Son, you've already been through so much. Do you want to do this surgery?"

Everyone turned to look at the boy. His face was still. Slowly, he nodded. His mother leaned close to hear him whisper, "Yes."

We left the room and began preparing to operate.

ONE DAY ELIAS WAS A NORMAL PERSON. He had graduated from high school and was living at home, taking college classes part-time while he worked to save money. He went fishing with his buddies, teased his little sister. Then he started coughing, and it didn't go away. Finally, he coughed up blood and was frightened enough to go to the doctor. Then, quite quickly, he became a different person: a young man dying of one of the most brutal cancers that we know.

Testicular choriocarcinoma affects young men, often in their twenties. The cancer starts in the testicle, then spreads so aggressively that it's rarely caught before it has moved through the bloodstream to the lungs, the liver, the brain. Elias coughed up blood because the cancer was in his lungs.

Here is the terrible part. Choriocarcinoma comes from germ cells—primordial cells in the testicle that could turn into many other kinds of cells. In this case, they turn into placental tissue. This means that the cancer does what placentas do: it burrows into tissue like a placenta would burrow into the wall of the uterus, and then it starts building blood vessels. When a placenta builds blood vessels, that means that the fetus inside can get nutrients from its mother's bloodstream. But when choriocarcinoma builds blood vessels, it just means that this cancer bleeds. So every time a new lesion popped up in Elias's body, it would burrow in—into his brain, into his lung—and begin to bleed ferociously.

To the neurosurgery team, this meant that Elias needed a brain scan any time his symptoms changed. If his right pupil dilated, or

his head flopped back because his neck had grown weak, or his lip
slumped, it could be a sign that a new lesion was bleeding into his
brain, putting pressure on his brain and brain stem. These lesions
needed to be dealt with quickly, because brain bleeds can kill a person quickly.

By the time I met Elias, he had been through two rounds of chemotherapy and had been admitted to our hospital for emergency
brain surgery. The first brain bleed damaged his cortex, and the surgery further damaged his brain. Quite simply, to get to a tumor in
the brain quickly, you have to cut through healthy brain tissue. The
outcomes are often poor. Patients who survive can be left severely
disabled from the combined effects of brain cancer and brain surgery.

We were actually trying to get Elias transferred to another hospital
where he could get whole-brain radiation in the hopes of stopping
the brain metastasis. But he had popped another bleed before he'd
even recovered from his first brain surgery enough for transfer, so we
were going in again.

ON MY NEUROSURGERY ROTATION, I would bicycle to the hospital around 4:45 a.m. I'd page one of the doctors and round with
him, going from room to room to see all the patients on our service.
We rounded quickly, and behind every door we opened there was
some new horror. We would often start with the young woman who
appeared perfectly healthy but could remember nothing. She had had
a brain infection that had required multiple surgeries, and was still in
the hospital in part because there was nowhere else to send her. Every
morning, we would shake her awake and ask her her name.

"I . . . I'm not sure," she would say. She seemed embarrassed.

"It's Nan," the doctor would say. "Your name is Nan."

"Oh, thank you!" she would say. "Nan." And then she'd go back to
sleep. Outside in the hallway, the doctor told me she probably wasn't
going to get any better. Behind another door, there was the man who
went hiking and dove head first into a shallow pool, arriving at our

emergency room unconscious with a massive bleed pushing his brain stem down against the base of his skull. There was the woman who was pushed from a moving car by her partner; she had been in the hospital for three weeks, and her head was still so swollen that her eyes were pressed shut and her face was unrecognizable. There was the thirty-eight-year-old mother who had a bad headache and then suddenly keeled over on her kitchen floor from an aneurysm. There was the junior high school teacher who cracked his skull on a sidewalk, the jogger who was hit by a truck. We would shrug on yellow gowns and gloves to see the brain cancer people, wraith thin, in isolation because their immune systems were trashed by the medicine. Our patients had big areas of their heads shaved where we'd cut into their brains, and thick black stitches arched across their skulls. Some were on ventilators in the ICU. Some were breathing on their own, but you had to rub their sternums hard or dig your fingernail into their nail beds to make sure they were responsive to the only stimulus they could still react to: pain.

Rounds made me face the consequences of our work. In the operating room I could focus on the problem at hand, follow each step, and even have a sense of accomplishment: We found the source of the bleeding! We sucked out the tumor! On rounds, I had to peel up the eyelids of the patients, gaze into their pupils, and think, *We did this*.

Many of our patients were young, especially the trauma patients. And many, especially those who hung on in states of semiconsciousness, were alone. There would be family at first, but gradually the rooms would empty, leaving these wounded people locked alone in whatever minds they retained. I would pass by their rooms sometime before dawn, rake my knuckles across their sternums until they startled, and then leave them alone again.

Eventually, they were all alone, except for Elias and the jogger. The jogger was my mother's age, but she had no children. She had gone out jogging on a Saturday morning and been hit by a truck. Her face split open at the eyebrow—a job for plastic surgery—and her brain smashed against the front of her skull. We had temporarily taken a bit of her skull off to relieve the pressure on her swollen brain, then stapled her skull back together when the swelling reduced.

I remember her husband in the emergency room right after the accident, sitting at her bedside and petting her arm, whispering to her. He was in his fifties, his kind face contorted with fear. I looked back at him as we rushed her toward the operating room. He had one hand over his eyes and he was watching us through the cracks in his fingers, like a child who could not believe what was happening.

The jogger survived her surgery, but she would never be the same. This time it wasn't so much the surgery's fault as the fault of her injury—she was badly concussed, and it was hard to say how fully she would recover. She could put words together coherently, but she couldn't remember where she was. Her husband would sit beside her bed and read her stories, or just gently hold her. He slept in her room, and would wake up to talk with us each morning when we rounded.

One afternoon I went in to check on the jogger's stitches, and her husband and I talked for a while as I used a soft brush to clean the dried blood from around them.

"Can you do the stitches on her face, too?" he asked. "She's always been pretty. I think she'll feel better if those are cleaned up a bit."

"Sure," I said. It was late afternoon and we were done with surgeries for the day. Golden light slanted in through the room. It was quiet in there, away from the beeping monitors of the nursing station. I took my time.

When I was done, the jogger did look better. The dried blood had made her face look freshly wounded, but now she just had the clean line of stitches and some swelling. Her husband smiled into her face. "That looks so much better!" he said. "Here, honey, look at this mirror. Look how pretty you are!" And he walked her gently over to the mirror by the sink, smiling into her reflection. The thick black stitches made a rectangle on the shaved left side of her head, and another jagged line of smaller stitches went from the middle of her forehead down through her eyebrow to her cheekbone. They stood close beside each other, with their fingers laced together.

"I'm pretty?" she asked him.

"You're beautiful," he said.

ELIAS'S SECOND SURGERY WENT SMOOTHLY. I headed down to the operating room along with the neurosurgeon and the nurse practitioner. We all scrubbed, washing our hands and arms for five minutes with strong antiseptic soap, and nudged through the swinging door of the OR backward, with our clean hands before us. The scrub nurse got us gowned and gloved, and the doctor requested Mozart.

We looked quickly at Elias's brain scans, which a nurse had pulled up on the computer screen in the OR. This new tumor was on the opposite side from the first one, so we would have to drill a new hole instead of going in through the same place we did for his last surgery.

"I think his family is pushing him," the nurse practitioner said.

"Yes," the doctor said. "I wouldn't choose this."

"They know he's dying?" the nurse practitioner asked.

"They've been told," the doctor said, "but I don't think they believe it."

Elias was anesthetized by the time we finished reviewing the scans. A little huddle of people was around him—the anesthesiologist at his head, gently pushing a tube down his throat and then moving away so we could get to his skull. It was already shaved, so the doctor began quickly—cutting through the skin with a scalpel, then drilling burr holes. There was no role for me in this surgery. Since we had to move quickly, I would only slow things down. I stood beside the nurse practitioner and watched. The doctor used a tiny rotating saw to connect one hole to the next, and we lifted away a rectangular portion of Elias's scalp. Underneath this was the dura mater—the thick outer layer of meningeal tissue that surrounded his brain. It was cloudy, like wax paper. Moving quickly, the surgeon cut through it and exposed the brain. The brain looked pink and perfect, shiny like candy. The tumor was deep inside. We cut down toward it, through the matter that held his memory of all language, his ability to kick a soccer ball smoothly across a lighted field at night, the shape of his mother's face. We found the bleeding tumor, and sucked it out through a tube.

I know it's awful to say it like that, because you probably want to imagine neurosurgery as this perfect science. You want it to be precise and technical, guided by benevolent machines. Sometimes it is like that. But the tube that sucked up the bloody mass in Elias's brain made the same sound you hear at the dentist when they suck saliva from the back of your mouth.

I LEFT THE HOSPITAL in a hurry after Elias's surgery. I pedaled hard uphill past the university and onto Manor Road, trying to shuck that hospital feeling. I wanted to leave Elias behind, to let him wake up with a freshly mutilated brain surrounded by his family, to let my mind let them alone. I breathed in the still-hot October air, and yanked up the leg of my scrubs when it caught on the gearshift. My scrubs ripped at the ankle. I breathed out and stood up to pedal harder. I was twenty-eight and alive, and I was going on a date.

I went home and changed into normal clothes, then biked back out to the Long Branch Inn. It was a blind date in the sense that all Internet dates are blind dates, so when I walked in from the sunny sidewalk I stood blinking a moment in the dim bar, unsure of whom I was looking for. A man stood up, and I walked to him, smiling.

I don't remember what we talked about that night, but I remember thanking god that he was funny. I described my neurosurgery rotation in the vaguest outlines; his mother was a nurse so he understood about how people want to leave those things behind sometimes. And, in his presence, I did. I was no longer the medical student on the neurosurgery service, but a live woman! We went outside and ate tacos that he had brought. When we got on our bicycles to go home, we realized that we lived just a few blocks away from each other.

I felt like a human again, that night. I was out of the hospital. I had a crush.

———

THAT HUMAN FEELING DIDN'T LAST LONG, though. In the morning, I discovered that Elias couldn't talk anymore. He couldn't move much of his body. He could understand language, and he could communicate by holding up one finger. His family was still all around him, reading, talking, praying. They wanted us to continue our efforts. They believed in miracles from God, and would hear no talk of gentling him toward death. The possibility of whole-brain radiation, if we could get him out of our hospital, sounded like hope to them, a pathway toward some miracle. I stood quietly beside the surgeon and realized what we had done to this nineteen-year-old boy who, we knew, was surely dying of his cancer.

If the neurosurgery team was Cerberus, the three-headed hound of Greek mythology that you pass on your way into hell, then I was the weakest head that month. I couldn't do much. I just sat quietly, attached to some complex devil but only watching as my patients— too desperate to refuse our knives, longing too badly to stay in any kind of world—passed by.

It is strange to move from that twilight world back into the world of the young and healthy and living. One day that week, I left the hospital early and drove out to a beautiful cool-water spring in the Hill Country with the man I had started dating. We lay in the sun in our swimsuits on a limestone rock, and when we swam, the cool water ran over our arms and legs. We rose easily and walked down a path through the cypress and pin oaks, and we kissed on a rock that was scattered with flowers. Fireflies flashed over the water, and like my patients, I wanted desperately to be in this world. His heart beat fast against me when we kissed, and when I touched him I felt like I was flinging myself toward life, life, any kind of life.

I WAS ASLEEP WHEN MY PHONE RANG at three in the morning the following week. It was Dr. Ijimo. "Well, Rachel, I guess you ought to come on down here, because we have an emergency craniotomy to do." I rolled out of bed, shrugged on my scrubs in the darkness of my bedroom, and drove to the hospital. The parking garage was empty enough for me to get a spot on the first floor, so I hustled into the bright-lit nighttime hospital and straight to the operating suite.

By the time I was scrubbed, Dr. Ijimo had already opened the patient's skull and was preparing to maneuver his instruments down through the brain. The patient was covered by a light blue surgical drape so all we could see was the top of his head, but I remembered the pattern of fresh cuts I saw along this skull. It was Elias.

We sucked out another bleeding tumor, and as we were closing up I turned to Dr. Ijimo.

"He consented to this?" I asked.

"Well, this time he was unconscious," the doctor said. "His parents consented for him."

I just stayed in the hospital after that surgery. It was almost time for rounds, and there was no point trying to get any more sleep. I went to the hospital cafeteria for coffee, and took it out to the crappy meditation garden next to the back parking lot. It was five a.m., and I could hear the garbage trucks unloading Dumpsters beyond the garden fence. I thought of calling somebody, but it was too early—nobody would be awake. So I sat by myself and waited for this bad night to roll over into day.

Elias had survived the surgery and was in the recovery room. He would go from there to the ICU, and in the afternoon we would check on him. I was already dreading it.

ELIAS DID EVENTUALLY LEAVE our hospital alive.

I saw him there again six months later; I was on the internal medicine team, and he had come in with his lungs full of blood. I could not believe he was still alive. He was still able to raise one finger, and he communicated like that, though mostly his parents were calling the shots. It was never clear exactly how much Elias understood.

I ran into the nurse practitioner from neurosurgery in the hall. "Did you see Elias?" she asked.

"Yeah," I said. "I can't believe it."

"I'm so sorry," she said. "I feel so awful about this, but he needs to die."

"I know," I said.

"They need to let him die. He must be doing it for them. He wants to protect them, he doesn't want to let them down, so he won't stop."

"It's awful," I said.

"Everybody feels awful," she said.

If Elias had been a few years younger, the situation would have been different. A provision of the Affordable Care Act makes hospice and palliative care available to children even when they and their families want to continue potentially curative treatment. When the hospice team comes on board, they bring doctors and nurses who are experts not only in treating pain and other symptoms from life-threatening diseases but also in talking about death and dying. The hospice team could have prepared Elias and his family, in the most compassionate way possible, to face the situation. All doctors should be able to do this, frankly, but somehow communication had broken down in Elias's case.

But because Elias was over eighteen, getting hospice care at the same time as curative therapy was not an option for him. Hospice couldn't come on board until he and his family were ready to stop trying for a cure. We on the medical team knew pretty darn well— though nobody ever knows for sure—that a cure was not forthcoming. But his family wanted us to be heroes, and we tried too long to play that role.

It was easier for us at that time to put the blame on his parents for clinging to his life. But the fact is, we kept on doing the surgeries, even though we knew each one would leave him more devastated.

His parents chose to continue, and so we picked up our knives and continued. At a certain point, we could have refused.

But the fact is, Elias did get a few more months of life. Maybe he relaxed when his mother touched his cheek. Maybe his pain was well controlled. And maybe he saw fireflies. I don't know what it's like to be that young and to be dying, but I do know that life can be very beautiful. And I understood, that year, why Elias and his family clung to it.

CHAPTER 17

I DO NOT LIKE TO USE THE BATTLE METAPHOR FOR CAN-
cer, but in my grandmother Olive's case there can be no other: she
was a soldier's wife and, in her own way, she fought. She had gone
to college and gotten her teacher's certification in her forties, just
years before she was diagnosed with breast cancer. Her teaching
career was precious to her: it was all her own. In all those years I
knew her, when she was on and off chemotherapy, she continued
teaching. She taught reading to public-school children with special needs. When the Corpus Christi Independent School District
wanted to recognize her for being their oldest teacher, she refused
to accept the award: "I don't want people to know how old I am,"
she said, patting her thin gray curls. "That's nobody's business."
When MD Anderson in Houston refused to give her targeted radiation for her bone metastases, she started flying up to Washington
for the treatments. When she woke up one morning and all of her
toenails had fallen out from the effects of chemo, she put on her
socks and shoes and went to school.

Olive could be terrifying to children. She claimed that my
brother and I read too much and were ruining our vision, so we
would flee to a brown corduroy chair on the upstairs landing of
her house and read away the afternoons of our Corpus Christi

family vacations, safely hidden. Olive wasn't much for negotiating the stairs. She would rule the house from her own recliner, delivering scathing commentary on Olympic ice dancing or on the many failures of her five children's husbands and wives. Her own husband—my grandfather Charles—took to the kitchen in his old age, cranking out beautiful pie at the holidays and gently spoiling my brother and me. He was the one with the wonderful stories of his years as a ranger in the National Parks Service. He had ranged over Yellowstone, the Smoky Mountains, and Grand Canyon National Park, keeping Olive and the kids in Park Service housing (much to Olive's disdain). In the years before, while he was a soldier stationed in Ethiopia, Spain, and Germany, they never lived on an Army base. Olive wanted to live in the cities; she wanted to be far from the kind of people she was raised among on a farm in Gonzales, Texas. She dressed beautifully, hoarding gowns and shoes and fancy purses that she bought at deep, deep discount. My grandfather, for his part, never told me stories about his years before the Parks Service. He had enlisted as a Marine at the outset of World War II, when country kids were in high demand as infantrymen because they already knew how to shoot. He fought in the Pacific, and was involved in the storming of numerous islands.

Grandpa mustered out of the Marines after the war ended, and worked odd jobs and studied dentistry before signing up again as an Army man. He was sent to officer school, and eventually retired as a major. Then he finished college and got his Parks Service job. Those were the stories he told me. Like how one day when they were living in Grand Canyon National Park the family woke up to find my seven-year-old uncle missing. The boy spent that day hiking all the way to the bottom of the canyon and back in slippers and a bathrobe. "I bet you could do that, too," my grandpa told me.

Olive could terrify a shopkeeper as well as a child. One summer when my brother was five, Olive was watching my mother fold up a pair of his underwear that had a hole worn in it.

"Where did you get those underwear?" she snapped.

"Sears," my mother said.

"Sears?" Olive asked, a glint coming into her eye. "Get in the car, Reta. We're taking them back."

"But I bought them a year ago, and I don't have a receipt," my mother said. "They're just worn out."

Olive had sniffed out a battle, though, and would not be swayed. "Those underwear are faulty," she said firmly. "We are taking them back."

"Yes, ma'am," my mother said.

So Olive drove my mother out to the Sears in Corpus Christi, where she proceeded to present the worn-out underwear to the poor gal at the service desk. "These underwear are faulty," she explained gently. "They have a hole." Olive got the underwear replaced, in the larger size that my brother now needed.

After my grandfather was diagnosed with Alzheimer's, my mother would send me out to the breezeway to listen to his stories as he smoked his pipe. So together we would pass the long afternoons, tending quietly to the rosebushes that he cultivated in the sandy soil. I loved these afternoons; I didn't realize until long after that we were probably both hiding from Olive.

TOP-NOTCH CANCER TREATMENT kept Olive going for a long time, but it could not make her live forever. When the cancer finally overcame her, she wanted no tranquilizers. She wanted to be as lucid as possible, in total control of the family until her final moments. When she could no longer take food or breathe on her own, she wanted to be kept alive by machines for as long as possible.

But we refused.

I don't know if this was wrong or right, but after so many years, the family could not take any more protraction of our matriarch's death. We kept her at home, where she was in turns gentle and vicious. She would quietly thank me for sitting at her bedside and reading aloud to her from *Reader's Digest* or the *National Enquirer*, then lay into my father and his brothers and the ghost of my grandfather, all of whom she blamed for penning her up, stealing her freedom, tying her to home.

"I could have been anyone," she said. "I was beautiful. Why did I have to marry that stupid Army man? There were dozens of men courting me." Then she would lie back on her pillow, waiting for me to offer her another sip of water.

"She forgets," my mother comforted me later. "She forgets how much she loved him; she forgets that if she hadn't married him, she wouldn't have you."

But Olive actually never forgot. She was lucid the whole time, and fought until she died. It was terrifying to see someone die who was so very lucid, so angry, and who refused to accept that she was dying. *No*, she seemed to say, *this wasn't it. This wasn't what I wanted at all.* Not the five children, not the life abroad and in gorgeous national parks, not the hundred pairs of shoes that she left in boxes in her house, which nobody could bear to clean out for nearly a year after her death, so they remained like a monument to her. Not the quiet granddaughter by her side, reading. *Not this, and certainly not death. I refuse!*

When she could no longer fight death, she fought us, the living symbols of everything that now seemed empty about the whole business of being human, and particularly of being a woman. She became an ungrateful mother, tethered to the bed of her suffering by pain she could no longer escape.

My father came home from tending to her one evening, and in his grief and his exhaustion he said, "If she could suck years out of my life so that she could live a little longer, I know she would." He was the eldest son.

"Oh Chuckie, no, no," my mother said, moving toward him. But I think she knew it was true.

———

IN MY OWN HOUSE TODAY, there are things that were Olive's. There is a brown leather footstool from Ethiopia, two fancy dresses, a pair of expensive sandals I wear in the summertime, and that old corduroy chair from her upstairs landing. It's still a great reading chair, and when I snuggle down into it these days I feel as safe as I did when I was a child—no longer safe from Olive, but safe near her. Or near enough, with the protective distance of mortality.

My brother planned to name his boat after her. Boats all have names, and so he knew when he bought a used boat that he would have to change the name. But changing a boat's name is bad luck, and like most sailors, Matt is loath to invite bad luck. To change the name to Olive Belle—including her middle name there—he would first have to find a maiden to pee on the deck. That's how, apparently, you cast away the bad luck.

We joked about how it would be hard to find a maiden in Southeast Alaska, and how we might have had to send up one of our baby cousins. Matt would shake his head and say, "Aw, I've got buddies who have kids. I bet one of 'em has a daughter." Dad suggested a Craigslist ad: *Looking for virgin to pee on boat.* But Matt figured that would get him arrested, or at least investigated.

When Matt finally did find his boat, the name it already had was glorious: the *Viking Rover.* So he kept that name, and I—imagining storms, anger, the fierce rage of a woman dying—was relieved. Olive can be a great protective spirit, but you never know when she might turn.

CHAPTER 18

IN THE SPRINGTIME OF MY THIRD YEAR OF MEDICAL school, I did a three-month rotation in internal medicine. For the final month, I was sent out to work in a private practice office in a wealthy Austin neighborhood. I arrived early Monday morning and introduced myself to the receptionist, who called back to Sara, the medical assistant, who led me through the clinic door into the back and showed me around while we waited for Doctor Houston. There were two doctors in this practice, so there were two sets of examination rooms, plus a procedure room where, as Sara explained, "they do all the laser hair removal."

"They do laser hair removal?" I asked.

"Yeah!" Sara said. "Doctor Houston does. And you can actually get an employee discount if you want to get it done here. I got a full Brazilian, and it's great."

"A full Brazilian?" I asked.

"Yeah!" Sara said. "But you can get whatever. Just the sides, or a little strip. You know."

"Oh cool," I said. I was not accustomed to discussing my pubic hair before eight a.m. in a professional setting. "Um, I think it might be kind of weird for that to be done by someone I work with, though."

"Oh, he's totally professional. He does it all the time," Sara said. "Here's a pamphlet."

I took the pamphlet and we moved on, past a suite of chairs designed for people to get electrode treatment for diabetic foot pain, past another set of exam rooms, and out toward the bathroom. In the hallway to the bathroom, there was a display case showing the high-protein diet regimen for sale through the office—you could have snacks and meals on this special diet delivered to your home.

"Dr. Houston actually did this diet himself," Sara whispered to me. "He lost fifty pounds. He looks great."

"Oh, great," I said.

We headed back down the hallway. "So what's up with the electrode chairs?" I asked.

"Oh, it's so awesome," Sara said. "You know how people with diabetes get all that pain in their feet? Well, we're the only clinic in the area where they can get this electrode treatment. Our patients love it. Dr. Houston tries to make it like a spa for them, because they have to come in three times a week for the treatments for six weeks. Some of them put cucumber slices over their eyes."

"Cool," I said. "Is that on insurance?" I asked, wondering who could afford to pay for eighteen treatments out of pocket.

"Oh, no," Sara said. "It hasn't been approved by the FDA yet. But Dr. Houston says it definitely will be."

As we passed back toward the exam rooms, sure enough, an older lady was relaxing in one of the chairs with her cane leaned up against the side and cucumber slices over her eyes.

"That's Mrs. Vandeem," Sara whispered. "She's a hoot."

Private practice was indeed different from training in a public hospital, but not for the reasons I expected. The patients mostly had what we call "bread and butter" medical issues: high blood pressure, low thyroid, flu. We saw some more complicated patients, and some cancer survivors, but it was a profound relief to practice in a space where everyone was well tended. Not only did they have full access to care but they also had every other social advantage that leads to health: money, fresh food, clean safe neighborhoods with space to exercise, job security. We could offer them the best medical care, and trust that they'd be able to do the rest. I loved the work. It was deeply satisfying to be able to use my training to help people; it was so clear.

Dr. Houston was great, too—the kind of smart, warm, no-nonsense doctor I'd like to have for myself. He would send me in to see the patients on my own, for a history and physical exam. Then I would report to him, and we'd go confer with the patient.

On my second morning in the clinic, I walked in to see a woman in her fifties with hypothyroidism. She looked up brightly as I walked in the door, but then her face darkened.

"Hi, I'm Rachel," I said, reaching out to shake her hand.

She did not extend a hand. "Who are you?" she asked.

"I'm the third-year medical student working with Dr. Houston. I'll just get started with you and then he'll join us."

"Do you have to?" she asked, frowning.

"Oh," I said. "No. If you don't want to see a student, you definitely don't have to."

"I'd rather not," she said.

"That's fine," I said. "I'll let Dr. Houston know you're waiting."

"Okay," she said.

I backed out of the room and closed the door behind me. I felt strangely ashamed, having intruded briefly into this woman's life and been repelled. In the three years I had been seeing patients, none had ever refused to see me.

This would happen almost every day in Dr. Houston's practice, and it never failed to make me feel bad. Of course, I know that patients have no obligation to see students, and I don't really want to see patients who don't want me there. But these patients, who had so much more protection than my St. Vincent's patients, and were so much healthier, were unlikely to be harmed by me. Why were they the ones who refused?

There was also a type of patient whom Dr. Houston didn't let me touch: his Botox patients. Botox is a commercial form of botulism toxin that is used to paralyze muscles. In patients with torticollis—a painful forced twisting of the neck—Botox can be used to relax the neck. It's also sometimes used in the esophagus to relax a chronically tight muscle. And, famously, it's used to reduce wrinkles on people's faces. Dr. Houston's patients were using it for the latter.

When a Botox patient came in, Dr. Houston would transform from a serious-faced doctor into a chatterbox, animatedly discussing the pros and cons of paralyzing various facial muscles. One patient insisted that he wanted his forehead so paralyzed that his eyebrows would be totally immobile. Another lamented that she couldn't make it to the Botox party this month—after-hours gatherings in the clinic where Dr. Houston would serve wine and multiple patients would come together to have their facial muscles chemically paralyzed.

When these patients would come in, I would just stand in the back and watch as Dr. Houston inserted the tiny needles into their skin. It was strange—I'd been allowed to do so many more invasive procedures, so why not Botox? It was a pure luxury transaction: patients paid to have a professional—a doctor—manage their beauty. There was no place for a student in this transaction.

THE EXCESSES OF LUXURY CARE I saw in Dr. Houston's office seemed mostly benign, but they made me think. Excess was not always benign, as I knew from my mother's story.

In 2000, when she was forty-six, my mother donated blood at the high school where she worked as a biology teacher. A few weeks later, she got a letter in the mail that said, on the top, "THIS IS NOT A LETTER TELLING YOU THAT YOU HAVE HIV."

Why would they write that? my mother thought, and her blood ran cold.

The letter said that her blood had tested positive for something called "non-A, non-B hepatitis," and that she should see a doctor. There were no details, but a memory floated up before my mother's eyes: years ago in the 1990s, something similar had happened. A doctor found something in her blood—she couldn't remember what—but then the second test for it was negative. He told her not to worry about it, and so she didn't.

But the doctor my mother found this time was worried. Knowledge about hepatitis C—the virus formerly known as non-A, non-B hepatitis—had progressed since the 1990s. Now, it was understood to be a virus transmitted from blood to blood (through blood transfusions, IV drug use, and sex that causes bleeding). The virus attacks the liver, gradually causing scarring. When the liver is so scarred that it can no longer clean the blood, patients go into liver failure and (in the absence of a transplant) die.

What was not entirely clear in the year 2000 was what my mother's particular chances of going into liver failure were. Her tests showed that her liver was not yet scarred, although she did have a high level of virus in her blood. And because hepatitis C had only been recognized as a distinct clinical entity since 1989, long-term studies of the outcomes of people infected with the virus were not yet available. Some people with the virus progressed to liver scarring, and some did not—they lived full lives and died of other things without ever being affected by the hepatitis C. The reasons for these different outcomes were not entirely clear.

So the doctor could tell my mother that she had this thing in her blood, and that it had the potential to make her horribly sick. To kill her. But she couldn't say if that would happen for sure, or when.

Sitting in the chair of the doctor's exam room, gripping my father's hand, my mother felt her body change. The body that had hopped on the back of my father's motorcycle and ridden through the Ozark Mountains in the autumn of 1978, had borne two children and held our hands walking through a hundred forests, gone to college and become a teacher, hammered nails into the roof of our house—suddenly her body could not be trusted. Suddenly it harbored a monster that could turn on her at any time.

The doctor was serious and calm.

"How did I get this?" my mother asked.

"It's hard to say," she answered. "The virus travels in the blood, so exposure to infected blood is how you get it. Were you ever a nurse or a health care worker?"

"No, but I worked for the Health Department in Montgomery County," my mother said.

"Any needle sticks or exposure to blood there?"

"No."

"Have you ever used IV drugs?" the doctor asked.

"No."

"What about any blood transfusions?" And my mother began to answer *no*, but then she remembered: there had been one. In the summer of 1983, after my mother gave birth to me, the doctor ordered a blood transfusion for her. She felt okay at the time, and hadn't fainted or anything. But the doctor said her blood counts were low, so she got the transfusion.

"Yes," my mother said, "there was one."

"And when was that?"

"Nineteen eighty-three." And that was the magic number, because between 1978 and 1989, scientists knew that some of the people getting liver infections after blood exposures were not getting them from hepatitis A or B—thus the term "non-A, non-B hepatitis"—but there was not yet a test for hepatitis C. And so my birth, and my mother's transfusion, fell into the high-risk window for infection with hepatitis C.

"So what do we do?" my father asked, and that was the question that led my parents from the world of the healthy into some twisty netherworld of treatment, where they would stay for many years, and from which they still have not recovered.

THERE WAS A NEW TREATMENT on the market, an experimental treatment, and my mother's doctor was eager to enroll her in a study so she could get this experimental medicine. It sounded very appealing: She would be at the forefront of medical care, taking a promising new drug that was not yet available to everybody. With my father's encouragement, she quickly agreed to join the study.

The first year of treatment was mundane and brutal. It consisted of pegylated interferon and ribavirin, two drugs that had a lot of the same effects as chemotherapy for cancer: my mother lost her hair, she was exhausted all the time, and she grew thin. But that year she was able to keep working. She'd drive around the bay to teach, then drive home and fall exhausted on the couch to sleep. She took to eating sweets—something I'd never known her to do—in an effort to keep weight on. Even so, she lost forty pounds. Her high school students, who only knew she was "taking chemo," made her hats. And so my mother, a longtime hat lover, was able to fully indulge herself. She wore straw hats, felt hats, and hats that her environmental-science students had decorated with little sharks and aquarium plants.

At home, she napped and apologized. "I'm sorry," she would say, just after vomiting. My father fretted around her in a cloud of inarticulate tenderness, then held her quietly on the couch when she was too nauseated to move. As she grew thinner, he feared that she would die, but he couldn't say it.

My brother and I were gone most of that year—he was at college, while I was away in the Spanish Canary Islands on a Rotary Club scholarship for high schoolers. I called home one day to suggest that we take a big family camping trip that summer, and my mother vaguely replied that she wasn't feeling too well that year, and wasn't sure she'd be able to make it.

"What do you mean?" I asked. "Not feeling well all year?" I was calling from my Spanish cell phone, sitting on some outdoor steps that led down toward a grocery store. I could see the ocean spread out below me, glittering, stretching away toward Morocco.

"I'm just a little weak," she said. "I'm taking some medicines. But I'm fine."

"Medicines for what?" I asked, beginning to cry.

"Don't cry, sweetie, don't cry. I'm fine. I'm really okay," she said.

"Medicines for what?"

"I have an infection in my blood, a virus. It isn't HIV. It isn't cancer. It's called hepatitis. I'm taking these new medicines all year, and they should make the virus go away."

"Mom."

"Don't worry, honey," she said. "I'm fine. I just don't want you to be too surprised when you get home, and I'm a little thinner and more tired than usual."

For the most part, I didn't worry. When I got home, I was tested for the virus. I was the last family member to be tested, and the one they'd been most worried about. Could I have been infected while breast-feeding, before I had an immune system of my own?* But I was not infected, and my mother wept beside me when I was back home and my results came in. I was surprised by her crying, and said "Mom. It's okay, I'm fine." Then I went off to college in the last months of her treatment.

The most mundane and brutal part of the whole ordeal was that it didn't work. The virus ebbed in her blood while she was on the drugs, but after the yearlong course was finished it came back as strong as ever. So all of that—the exhaustion and nausea, the weeping, the fear—all of it had been for nothing.

My father could not quite release his fear, and began to hold her more closely. He tried to keep her from driving at night, or in the rain. Unable to control the virus that threatened his wife's life, he began to try to control the things he could.

TEN YEARS LATER, I studied hepatitis in medical school. By that time, in 2010, we knew a fair amount about the different subtypes of hepatitis C, and about the relative risk of progression to liver scarring. We knew about the natural history of the disease and the molecular mechanisms that lead to liver damage. And we knew the epidemi-

---

* Hepatitis C is not spread in breast milk, but breast-feeding moms with the virus have to be careful about dry or cracked nipples, which can bleed.

ology: about one in two hundred Americans had hepatitis C. Rates were highest in the prisons, where IV drug use, rape, and consensual unprotected sex were common. (Hepatitis C is sometimes considered a sexually transmitted disease even though rates of sexual transmission are extremely low; sex that causes bleeding can transmit it.) So hep C had become one of those stigmatized conditions: an illness of poverty, depravity, immorality.

Stigma works in a funny way. My mother says that every random health care worker feels entitled to ask her how she got it. She doesn't look like the patient they expect—a burnt-out IV drug user or a former prisoner. And she could protest her innocence, but the whole paradigm offends her, so she usually says, "I'm sorry, but that's none of your business."

My mother has friends who have been to prison, family members who have suffered from addiction, and has lived under the poverty line herself. She knows that nobody deserves to suffer as she has.

My mother's disease, however, is likely related to the illness of those thought not innocent. In one lecture during my second year of medical school, the professor described the history of hepatitis C. "In the 1980s," he said, "we solicited blood donations from prisoners in Huntsville. The prisoners were an easy source of blood, which we desperately needed. But at that time, hep C was already rampant in the prisons, and we didn't know it. So in the 1980s, untold numbers of people in the Houston area were infected from transfusions of blood that had been taken from the prisons."

I sat there in the classroom, stunned. *My mother was one of those people*, I thought. She gave birth in Conroe, a half hour from Houston and a half hour from the prison in Huntsville. There's no way to know for sure, but the blood that infected her very likely could have come from the prisons.

It is no longer legal to solicit blood donations from prisoners. The practice was not only unsafe but also coercive. I cannot help but think, however, that the brutality of prison has affected my family just as it has so many others. If we were not incarcerating so many people; if prisoners had access to condoms; if rape were effectively prevented in the prisons . . . perhaps my mother would not have had to suffer so much.

MY MOTHER'S SECOND ROUND of hepatitis treatment was not mundane, but cruel. It began in 2011, in my third year of medical school, with another experimental treatment. Her liver was still healthy, but the possibility that the virus would one day kill her scared my father so much that Mom agreed to the treatment.

When she called to tell me about it, I was working on the internal medicine service. Just that week, I had seen a patient dying of liver failure from hepatitis C. He had lain in his hospital bed, his belly swollen and skin yellow, his arms and legs thin. He was on medications to prevent the sudden bouts of psychosis that poisoned blood can cause, but no medication could control the sweet stench that filled his room. The nurses rushed in and out, hardly able to bear it.

"You'll never forget that smell," my resident told me. "That's liver failure."

So when Mom said she was going to take the treatment, I agreed.

It was two medicines this time, to be taken for nine months. One had to be digested with fifteen grams of fat. And so, nauseated as she was, she had to find ways to consume forty-five grams of fat per day, for each round of medication. She ate bagels with cream cheese, ice cream, cheesecake. But she could hardly bear to swallow food, and so we tried to find ways for her to get the fat in with the fewest number of bites. Eventually, we found a kind of full-fat yogurt that has enough fat in a single serving, and my brother would make road trips to Austin to buy the yogurt for her.

The medicines made her thin, nauseated, and weak. Her hair thinned, her body changed. Her immune system was beaten down to a level where she couldn't go into public without a mask on. She became severely anemic, and when her blood counts got so low that she was short of breath, the doctors would order a transfusion. She began walking with a cane, and carrying a lightweight camping chair so that she could sit down suddenly if she needed to. When I went home for holidays, my father would meet me at the door and cook me a steak with red peppers, while my mother lay on the couch and smiled up at me. With my mother disabled by chemo and myself away at medical school, my father and brother, the carpenter and the fisherman, had become the primary caretakers of our family.

Things got pretty bad at home. My parents, who had always flirted and kissed in front of us, were no longer touching. My dad started smoking again, and would sit up nights in the living room alone. They moved out to Montgomery to be closer to specialists in Houston, and so—isolated out there in the country—their lives revolved around my mother's care.

Then, on the morning of the test for my ob-gyn clerkship, my brother called.

"Hey, sis," he said.

"Pearson," I said.

"Hey."

"Hey."

"So," he said. "I'm at the hospital with Mom. She wants to talk to you."

I sat down, while he passed her the phone. "Hi, Rachel," she said. "Listen, I'm okay."

"You're in the hospital."

"Well, I fainted in the bathroom last night, and your brother brought me in. They think my heart stopped."

"Your heart."

"I'm okay," she said again.

"Your heart stopped."

"Well, I'm okay. They're going to put in a pacemaker."

"You're in Houston?"

"I'm at the Woodlands. I'm okay."

"Okay, I'm on my way," I said. And she tried briefly to prevent me from coming, but her surgery was scheduled for that afternoon and my father was out of state, and I could not let her and my brother go through that alone. I knew she would be okay, but I could not let Matt sit out in the waiting room alone while she was in surgery. So I called to cancel my exam—no problem—and picked up barbecue on my way to Houston. With the hospital familiarity of an upper-level medical student, I climbed into my mother's hospital bed to give her the first big hug she'd had since fainting. My brother was sitting beside her, pale and worried. After a while, we walked out to the parking lot together, and he finally ate something, and finally cried.

"She screamed," he said. "When she fell. And I heard this noise, her falling. I thought she was dying." He had helped her out to his pickup truck and driven to the hospital with his flashers on.

Mom's heart had stopped at least twice—when she fainted at home, and again in the hospital. This is not a common side effect of the medications. It was complex, having something to do with her anemia and maybe something to do with an abnormal heart rhythm that had never been exposed before.

I knew how easily she could have died. She could have hit her head on the shower floor when she fainted, and bled into her brain. Her heart might not have started up again. She was out in Montgomery, in the house my father built off a dirt road that leads off another dirt road that is still a twenty-minute drive to the nearest hospital.

The pacemaker surgery made a small scar on her chest. The machine is there today, ready to throb out an electrical pulse if her heart should stop.

WHEN MY MOTHER WENT for her first round of blood tests after finishing treatment again, she was told that the treatment had failed. The virus was back. She kept the news between herself and my father for several weeks, then told my brother and me.

I was so angry.

"Don't you hate medicine?" I asked her. "You must. That doctor put you on all these experimental drugs, and your heart stopped, and nothing. No cure. Two years out of your life. Nothing."

But she didn't hate medicine, or she wouldn't tell me that she did.

When my mother gave birth to me, she was uninsured. She and my father and brother were living in that trailer in the woods in Montgomery, and he was working construction jobs for nine bucks an hour. They paid out of pocket for the birth, and for the transfusion that infected her. Obstetricians no longer routinely do transfusions on women with low blood counts after birth, unless they have symptoms such as a racing heart or lightheadedness. The practice is considered unnecessary, and too risky, so women are given a chance to recover and to gradually produce their own new blood. The transfusion that infected my mother was likely unnecessary: an excess of care, even though she was uninsured at the time.

But it was when she was fully insured that the real excess began. The first experimental treatment would have cost twenty thousand dollars a month without their insurance. The second would have been even more. At that time, we didn't even tell St. Vincent's patients about treatment for hep C. There was no way they could afford it. And that was sad, but some part of me also breathed a sigh of relief that they would be spared it.

And so when I saw the insured patients at Dr. Houston's office getting a little bit of "extra" medicine, it didn't feel benign to me. Everything that had happened to my mother felt so unnecessary: the transfusion, the failed treatments, the pacemaker, the fear of death that had fallen over everyone in our family and which we could not shake. Medicine had caused this.

LAST YEAR, WHEN MY MOTHER AND FATHER were camping in Idaho, my father got the idea that they should go to the Mayo Clinic. He sort of begged my mother to go. "What if something has changed?" he said. "Maybe there's something new."

My mother was no longer eager to try anything new. She no longer believed that it was good to be at the forefront of medicine, with access to the newest and best drugs. But she consented to call Mayo, mostly because she figured she wouldn't get an appointment anyway.

Yet she did, just a week later. And so my parents, the carpenter and the retired high school teacher, walked into the cathedral-like entryway of the most elite hall of American medicine, that top-level clinic that caters to the wealthy of the United Arab Emirates but does not accept poor patients with Medicaid. Finally, they had the kind of lives deemed worthy of care at the pinnacle of American medicine. A pianist was playing in the foyer.

The first day there, my mother had blood tests and underwent a new kind of liver ultrasound. Her appointment with the gastroenterologist was on day two. When he walked in, he was smiling.

"Well, good news," he said. "You don't have hepatitis."

"Yes I do," my mother said.

"Nope," he said. "You don't."

"I am sure that I do," my mother said.

"Nope," he said.

"What?" my father said.

The latest round of blood tests had shown that there was no detectable virus in her blood. The doctors couldn't explain—and they still can't—why it showed up right after her treatment and then disappeared.

And there was a final irony: the doctors at Mayo said that they would not have treated her. Even given the limited knowledge back in 2000, the best evidence suggested that my mother would never have been harmed by the virus. They would have just reassured her, and sent her out to live her life with occasional blood tests and liver ultrasounds.

So the virus is gone, and the whole ordeal was probably unnecessary. Unnecessary medicine stopped my mother's heart.

The rest of my family has taken her cure as a miracle, but I remain suspicious. I badger my mom about her follow-up tests, even though she's been disease-free for a year. She walks freely on the beach now, does water aerobics, hikes through the mountains with my dad. When we talk on the phone, she eventually starts identifying birds that she sees in the yard around her, and at that point I know it's time to hang up. All this is indeed like a miracle, when I remember her thirty blood transfusions and her years of illness, when I remember my patient dying of liver failure, and how desperately I wanted Mom to be free from that. My mother laughs again, and I hope that she and my father are recovering the kind of peaceful love they had before all this fear entered their lives.

CHAPTER 19

I RETURNED TO GALVESTON AS PLANNED IN AUGUST, after finishing my third year of medical school. I began taking courses at the Institute for the Medical Humanities again, and was made a junior director at St. Vincent's. I would become a full director in April, and serve in that position for a year before returning to just being a regular volunteer.

As a junior director, I started working on patient assistance—coordinating our patients' applications to pharmaceutical companies for free or reduced-price medications. Vanessa was one of the patients I was working with.

I first contacted Vanessa on the phone, to let her know that we needed a copy of her driver's license to send along with a patient assistance renewal request. The medication she needed was a controlled substance—Xanax—that we did not routinely prescribe at St. Vincent's. So, I hadn't known that it would require proof of ID. Vanessa was on her way home from the clinic when I called, but she turned around and drove back onto the island.

"I'm so sorry you had to drive all the way back here," I said, opening the door to the House for her. Our last patient was just leaving, and the outside doors were already locked. I felt annoyed on Vanessa's behalf; a real clinic, I was thinking, would have somebody who knew how to handle these things.

"Oh I know," she said. "The paperwork is a lot. Don't you worry." And she reached out and patted my shoulder.

VANESSA WAS BORN IN LOUISIANA, and she met her husband Jimmy there. Jimmy is her second husband. Her first, the father of her three daughters, was a mean drunk. When Vanessa finally left him, it was in the pickup truck of her second husband, Jimmy. She loves Jimmy, but Jimmy doesn't want her to work. He says it's too hard on her body.

Vanessa worked construction jobs most of her life. She was a pipe fitter, a welder, and even a foreman on some jobs. Being a woman foreman wasn't easy; you always had to prove yourself. But Vanessa was both tough and strong. These days, she looks down at her rounded body and laments the loss. "You should've felt my biceps, hon," she says. "They were so strong."

Vanessa kept working for a while after she married Jimmy, even though the two of them could've gotten by on Jimmy's income from his job at a refinery. Then Vanessa was hit by a truck on the highway just outside her home, and her back was so messed up that she could no longer stand for long periods. Construction was out. She tried working for a while in a laundromat, and for a while in a grocery store, but the pain got to her. And anyway, Jimmy liked having her at home. A time or two when we were talking, he would call and her voice would turn Louisiana-sweet while she told him she was with the doctor. Vanessa and Jimmy were uninsured, but they owned a house and were able to make the mortgage every month. Mostly, they just had to pay the household bills, plus food for the pets and for themselves. Their house was unscathed by Ike. There was never any extra money, and a time or two the lights were shut off, but usually there was just enough to get by.

Once, during a psychiatry night visit for Vanessa's anxiety, my mind wandered away while she was describing her travails with the house: they had to refinance the mortgage, but got a high rate because the place was zoned industrial. Pieces of concrete were pushing up through the ground all over the property as the land seemed to settle. Vanessa pried up one of the concrete coverings to find an underground tank, and her cousin, an oil-plant worker, tested it and found that it was full of old gasoline. The property was on top of an abandoned gas station. He estimated five hundred gallons of gas, with just a skin of water on top. Vanessa began to cry as she described the stress of all this—not only from the mortgage costs, but also the fear that the property was not safe for herself, or her plants and animals. "And Jimmy," she said. "He's been sick ever since we moved out there. I think it's affecting him."

I was sitting on a chair in a corner of the room while the psychiatrist faced Vanessa. The encounter had been dragging on, and it was late. This was not the first long story I'd listened to that night. I felt a kind of skepticism slipping through my mind. What was all this business about mortgages and chemicals? Couldn't we just get her medication and go home?

Then the psychiatrist turned to me. "Isn't that awful?" he said. "They've basically already paid for this property three times over." I could tell he was completely engaged with Vanessa's story and empathized with her. He's an older psychiatrist. He's listened to thousands more stories than I have, and he is not tired of listening at all.

"Oh, it's awful," I said, feeling a little ashamed of myself. I remembered what I had been learning in graduate school: doctors tend to rush out of encounters when we feel uncomfortable. Instead, we should slow down and ask more questions, work to build a relationship.

So, over time, I did. I made Vanessa my patient. I learned that she kept her plants in pots because she worried about the chemicals in the ground. She had lemons, peaches, plums, tomatoes, eggplant. When I saw her in the clinic over the next few months, the encounter always wrapped up with us swapping gardening stories: How she had to move her eggplants into the kitchen because of the frost. How my kale just wouldn't quit, but all my tomatoes gave up the ghost. How a mole got into her house inside one of the potted plants, and she had to hunt it down and kill it. I would get her prescriptions signed and we'd hug, and she'd be on her way. It was no longer a chore to care for her.

Then one day Vanessa came in sad, because one of her daughters had been arrested.

I told Vanessa how sorry I was. Vanessa pulled out her cell phone to show me a picture of her daughter, who was nineteen years old, thin, and smiling in a black one-shoulder dress. It was hard to imagine her in jail. "Oh," I said. "She's beautiful."

"Yes she is," Vanessa said. "She surely is." She flipped to a picture of Jimmy with her daughter in the living room of their house. Jimmy had a cigarette in his hand, and Vanessa's daughter was laughing with her mouth open. The walls behind them were unpainted plywood, like the walls of the trailer addition my father had been building that summer in 1981 when he sawed his fingertip off.

AFTER I BECAME A STUDENT DIRECTOR, I passed Vanessa's care on to other students. But we would always hug when we saw each other, and swap a story or two. She showed me pictures of her dogs, and would occasionally text me a photo when she harvested fruit from her potted lemon tree. I still called her on the phone to help manage her patient assistance prescriptions, and sometimes we would linger on the phone just catching up. It was one of those lopsided relationships that happen in the clinical world: we both cared about each other, but I knew the intimate details of her life while she knew very little about mine. For Christmas, she gave me a pair of earrings she had made from the tail feathers of her macaw. We laughed again over the story of Jimmy and her evacuating from Hurricane Ike with the macaw in their truck.

So I was surprised, but not shocked, when Vanessa called me one Sunday night. She had never called me before. "Rachel, you have to help me," she said. "They told Jimmy he's got cancer, and I don't know what to do."

Jimmy had come into St. Vincent's that Saturday, short of breath. He'd had a bad cold a couple of weeks ago, but then the cough lingered. On Thursday he began to feel short of breath, and Friday night he woke up choking for air. At St. Vincent's, Dr. Beach had listened to his lungs and heard fluid in them, so—fearing pneumonia—he sent Jimmy to the ER. With Jimmy's long smoking history, pneumonia could knock him out.

The ER doctors were probably worried about a pulmonary embolus—a clot in the lung—because they did a CT of Jimmy's chest. There was a pocket of fluid, but behind the pocket was a large, solid tumor.

As I listened to Vanessa, I suddenly felt stricken. On my internal medicine rotation the year before, I had learned that a new study— the low-dose CT scan—was effective at detecting lung cancer early enough to treat it and to extend life. Whereas a chest X-ray could only detect later cancer, and a full-dose CT could increase cancer risk from the radiation, a low-dose CT used minimal radiation and had been shown to be a cost-effective screening tool for long-term smokers. If Jimmy had been insured, his doctor almost surely would've recommended the low-dose CT. But I wasn't sure if we had even offered it.

I had, at times, refrained from telling my St. Vincent's patients what the standard of care would look like. I didn't talk with my hepatitis C patients about treatment (though I often tried to find funding for annual ultrasounds to screen them for liver cancer), and I had never offered the low-dose CT to a St. Vincent's patient. It would cost around $250 out of pocket. Vanessa and Jimmy just might have been able to swing it, if anybody had brought it up.

The UTMB doctors admitted Jimmy, gave him antibiotics, and put a tube in his chest to drain the fluid off of his lung. He got a biopsy of the tumor, which showed small-cell lung cancer, an aggressive type most common in smokers. When he was stable, he was discharged. He was not started on chemotherapy, or offered other cancer care. So Vanessa took Jimmy home and made him some dinner that he didn't eat, then set him up in their bedroom with the remote control. She cried until he went to sleep, then called me. How was she going to make sure Jimmy's cancer got treated? He couldn't have been sent home just to die.

There I was, in my own comfy bedroom on a Sunday night, with my dog sleeping under the desk, and a patient I cared for very much asking for my help in a desperate time. I didn't know what to do, but I did the only thing I could think of.

"Can you meet me at St. Vincent's tomorrow at one?" I asked.

"Yes," she said.

"Okay. Bring all your financial information, and we'll see what we can do."

I was struck then, as I am now, by the inadequacy of this response. With Jimmy newly diagnosed with an aggressive lung cancer, Vanessa should have been able to focus on the deeper questions that cancer makes us face: how to care for her husband, how to reckon with her own fear of his death, how to support him in having a meaningful life in the face of his diagnosis. All of these questions were somewhere in the mix, but at this moment they were obliterated by the question of how he could afford to get treatment.

My own response, too, had become bureaucratic. This could be a time for me to learn how to support a patient through fear and grief, but instead I would learn how to apply for financial assistance. Could this be what good doctoring is about? I downloaded the forms I could find online for UTMB financial assistance, and then I thought again of Vanessa, still likely awake in her house across the bay. Staring at my computer screen, I thought, *This can't be doctoring. This isn't it at all.*

In times of peril and grief, some distraction can be healthy. But in Vanessa's case, the bureaucratic intricacies of applying for financial assistance would distract her for too long. If Vanessa's most trusted advocate was a more experienced doctor, he or she might have seen the writing on the wall and taken time to ask Vanessa about her fear of death, or counsel her that Jimmy might not survive treatment anyway. But I was just a student.

Jimmy would die, and very quickly. And Vanessa would not be ready for his death in any way.

ST. VINCENT'S HOUSE was calm on Monday afternoon. A few patients were waiting to see their nurse practitioner at the nurse-managed day clinic, and one woman left with a grocery bag full of food from the food bank. The ladies said that Vanessa and I could use the chapel, so when she showed up we headed back there.

The financial assistance people at UTMB had given Vanessa an application to file for assistance with the bill from Jimmy's initial care. It needed to be returned within ten days of his discharge. So we started there.

If I were in Vanessa's situation, I would be at a loss. My finances are in order, but they aren't documented. Vanessa, however, had applied for assistance from social services before. She knew the drill, and so she carried a big manila folder into the chapel that held everything we needed: pay stubs, tax returns, a copy of their mortgage agreement, their car loan, their marriage license—everything. We spread the forms out all over the chapel, and they covered the chairs and half the floor. I used the St. Vincent's copier to make the copies she needed, and then we put it all in an envelope, with signatures, and mailed it off. It took about two hours.

This paperwork was not designed to secure care for Jimmy moving forward. Rather, it was only to help with the initial bill from UTMB. So I called Dr. Beach to see if he would sponsor a Casebook application for Jimmy, asking UTMB to take him on for unfunded cancer care. Dr. Beach was happy to sponsor the application, but warned me that it was unlikely to be accepted.

I knew he was right. Casebook had not accepted any St. Vincent's patients that I knew of, and the policies for acceptance were public but vague. UTMB could consider not only the severity and nature of the disease, but also whether the disease or treatment would offer "educational benefit" to students, residents, and fellows. This means that patients with unusual diseases, or who need procedures that the residents and fellows must complete for their training, may be more likely to be accepted. There is actually an acronym for this in the surgery world: RANDO, or "resident ain't never done one." RANDO cases are more likely to get taken on.

So, filling out the Casebook application was also uncomfortable for me. Jimmy would not be judged on whether he was a particular human being, who cared for his wife and their pets and his stepchildren. Instead, he would be judged on whether his suffering could be made useful for someone like me.

THE CASEBOOK APPLICATION was supposed to be approved or denied within two weeks. It was denied, but that didn't end up mattering because Jimmy got short of breath again, and Vanessa took him to a hospital in Houston where he was admitted through the emergency room.

He lingered there for three weeks, mostly on life support. He never got chemotherapy because he was never well enough for his body to sustain it. Vanessa would call or text every couple of days.

"He's on antibiotics again," she said one day.

"Now they've put him on a ventilator," a week later.

"I can't get this nurse to pay attention to him. He's bleeding out of everywhere, and the chucks on his bed are full of blood, and I can't get anyone to help. They don't treat uninsured people right in these hospitals," she said, and texted me pictures of a blood-soaked dressing on Jimmy's chest. His skin looked dark and unnatural; it looked like death.

So I wept on the phone a day later when Vanessa told me that the doctors wanted to pull the ventilator and let Jimmy die, but I was not surprised that he was dying. "I can't do it," she said. "He never got chemo, and now they just want to give up. I can't do it!"

The next day she said the same thing, and asked me what she should do. She was angry at the doctors for making her decide; she didn't want to feel, years later, like she had killed her husband.

I was still just a student, but I gave her the best advice I could. "I know how much you love him, Vanessa," I said. "I know how much you hate to see him suffering. I'm sorry you have to make this decision, but I know that you are the only one who can make this decision from a place of love."

"I know," she said. "I know."

They pulled the ventilator, and the next morning Jimmy died.

VANESSA GRIEVED FOR A LONG TIME. She was also afraid, blindsided by the bills from Jimmy's death. There was a $17,000 bill from UTMB, and $325,000 for his three-week stay in the intensive care unit in Houston. Vanessa was still unemployed, and terrified that she would lose the final thing that—now that Jimmy was gone—stood between her and abject poverty: her house. So there was the grief, and on top of the grief there was fear.

Over time, she drew on her inner resources. She sought retraining in work skills that she could use despite her persistent back pain and the problems in her feet. She got two part-time jobs, and when she became a manager at a local store she even got insurance, so she is no longer a St. Vincent's patient. Neither of Vanessa's jobs are high paying, but she has kept up with the mortgage and is in her home.

When I asked her if she thought Jimmy would have been better off if he hadn't been a St. Vincent's patient, Vanessa says no. Sometime during Jimmy's illness, a doctor comforted Vanessa by telling her that there was nothing she could have done. Lung cancer is aggressive and hard to catch. There is no way she could have stopped it. Vanessa takes comfort in this.

When I return to the question that Susan McCammon once asked me about Mr. Rose—"What do you wish you would have done differently?"—I sometimes wish that I had made sure Jimmy at least

knew about the low-dose CT, so he could have made his own decision. He probably wouldn't have gotten it anyway, with money so
tight. But he could have made that choice.

Sometimes I wish I had talked with Vanessa about hospice. A more
experienced advocate—a doctor—might have suspected that Jimmy
was going to die quickly. If he had had hospice, he might have died
not only more comfortably but with much less of a financial burden
passed on to Vanessa.

On the other hand, hospice is not designed to be forced on the
poor. Hospice should be a choice—one offered to patients when they
have exhausted the available treatment options, or when they know
that treatment is not an option they want to pursue. Between the
time Jimmy left UTMB and the time he checked into the hospital
in Houston, no doctor was talking to him about his disease. He had
no regular primary care provider, who would know him and his
needs and be there to counsel him about hospice. Rather, he had St.
Vincent's, where a rotating cast of volunteer students and doctors
would tend to him, and where it routinely took three weeks to get
an appointment.

More than anything else, I wish Vanessa and Jimmy had had a
more experienced advocate than me. Not because I did a bad job. I
did a good job for someone at my level. But I was just a student, and
there were many things I did not know. They deserved, as everyone
does, a doctor.

CHAPTER 20

DERMATOLOGY NIGHT AT ST. VINCENT'S IS NOT A BOTOX party. In fact, dermatology night at St. Vincent's cured me of my haughtiness about dermatology in general. Having observed how medical students grow progressively more taut and attractive as soon as they decide to go into dermatology—eventually progressing from being pale schlubs like the rest of us to being fine, glowing specimens, almost as good-looking as the physical therapy students who regularly humiliated me at group exercise classes in the UTMB gym—I had nothing but disdain for dermatology. One friend suggested I go into it, and I said, "Pshaw! I want to be a *doctor*." But dermatology night at St. Vincent's was mostly cancer prevention and cancer care.

It was also a good time to do procedures, like biopsies. One derm night when I was volunteering as a junior director, I pulled a chart and began looking it over with a physician assistant (PA) student who was at the clinic for the first time. The patient had recently been diagnosed with hepatitis C, the same virus my mother had. She was a smoker, and had a history of small growths on her skin, including her face, that needed to be removed and biopsied. At this appointment, we planned to biopsy a spot on her leg that had grown rapidly in the last few months.

"This will be a good case for you to see," I said to the PA student.

"Watch how we do the biopsy, so next time you can do one." The PA student and I discussed the hep C—though I didn't mention why I knew so much about it—and went over strategies for talking with patients about quitting smoking. Then, we called the patient back into an exam room.

She was a thin woman in her fifties. She greeted us coolly, and we arranged ourselves in one of the smaller exam rooms. The patient sat in a straight-backed plastic chair, and I sat on the rotating doctor's stool. The PA student, clearly trying to take up as little space as possible, wedged herself into a corner chair behind me.

As we talked, the woman began to tell us about all the student volunteers who had messed up her care in the past: a student who swiped three times at a mole on her eyelid before removing it, one who was plain rude to her, and one who dabbed cautiously at a small growth on her face instead of freezing it off quickly and smoothly like she should have. The growth came back, bigger. She felt ugly.

By the end of these stories, she was crying. "This is humiliating," she said. "I have worked my whole life, and still. I have to sit through this. This is real," she said, looking at me. There was an accusation in her eyes, a conviction that I was on the far side of a chasm I could never understand. "This is what it's like," she said, "when nobody gives a shit about you."

I almost protested. I wanted to say, "I give a shit about you." I wanted to tell her that I came from a working-class family, and I'm not so far from understanding what it's like to be shut out. She didn't know me.

But how could I protest now, in the fourth year of my medical education? I was different. No amount of research, and no shared experience, could teach me what it was like to be a free-clinic patient—or to be this particular woman. The white coat was on me. The knife that would cut into her skin was waiting in the hallway supply closet, and it would be in my hand.

Anyway, this patient had good reason not to trust me. I believed the stories she was telling about student screwups. I was, after all, preparing to do a shave biopsy on her leg with a small blade that I'd never used before. I knew it was going to be awkward. There was a chance I'd mess it up, just like the students in the past. I also thought of the student sitting behind me, and wondered what she must be thinking about our clinic.

Some part of me is grateful when a patient can just tell it like it is. Charity care patients most often keep silent when they know their care is inadequate. If they made us angry, and we stopped seeing them, they would have nowhere else to go. So whenever a patient finds it in herself to complain, I remember all the other patients who are going through the same thing, but don't say a word.

Instead of protesting, I stalled. I knew the woman had a good job, and might be eligible for care through the ACA health exchange. So I brought that up. "I want you to get the best care," I said. "And I know that St. Vincent's isn't always the best care. Have you thought about checking out the health exchange? Especially with your hepatitis, you might be able to get better care."

She hadn't. And she wasn't planning to. She'd already been rejected by the county and by UTMB, and she had no faith in the federal government to get her better care. She said she already knew she couldn't afford it, even with the subsidy. And, finally, she had seen friends go through intensive, and unsuccessful, drug therapy for hepatitis. She wanted no part of that special suffering.

"This is not my fault," she said. Her voice was firm even though she was still crying. "There is nothing else that I need to do."

I was silent for a minute. I could feel how deeply she didn't trust me, and how that lack of trust made my advice on the health exchanges useless. The best thing for her care would be to get her insured, and into the office of a regular primary care doctor. But until she trusted me, my advice wouldn't make a difference in her health.

She narrowed her eyes and shook her head. I wanted to flee.

I breathed in deeply and made myself stay. The PA student actually did flee the room, mumbling about bringing a tissue. Handing a tissue to patients is the official medical response to patients' crying.

They actually teach you, in medical school, to give a tissue to crying patients, and I've seen full-fledged doctors literally run out of the room in pursuit of tissues. It's not clear if they're running for the tissue, or away from the patient, but they clearly are trying to "do something."

Tissue accepted, we sat quietly a little longer.

"I'm sorry," I ventured.

"Just take care of this for me," the woman finally said. "That's all I want. I just want you to do this, and then I want to go home."

So, I agreed to take care of the one small thing that I could, and we left the room. The PA student was wide-eyed. "That was intense," she said.

I looked at her, remembering that I was supposed to be teaching. "Well," I said, "I think we have some work to do to establish trust."

"Uh, yeah," she said, with a tone that suggested, *No fucking joke, you bozo. This woman hates us.*

I DID NOT LEARN to do all of my procedures on patients. There was the MUTA-GTA, where we learn to do genital exams on standardized patients, and then there was the annual St. Vincent's volunteer orientation, where a hundred and fifty brand-new medical students learn to draw blood—on one another.

All of us directors liked running the orientation sessions, which happened once or twice a week throughout the fall. We liked showing off the clinic, and telling about its history, and preparing junior students to worship us as gods. The medical hierarchy has a way of promoting hero worship, and we were delighted to find that, as fourth-year students, we were finally eligible. When I introduced a whistle to orientation—*Okay, the director blows the whistle, and then all the first-years run to the next station!*—even the grumpiest directors began signing up to take orientation shifts.

Practicing blood draws was the last part of orientation, and it was what really brought the students in. I would stand at the front and walk through the steps of the blood draw—find a vein, get the arm ready, swipe it with alcohol, put on a tourniquet, brace your hand, then *stab the crap out of your patient* at a thirty-degree angle to the skin—ha ha, just joking, quickly insert the needle at a thirty-degree angle—*don't jump if they scream*, put on the vacuum tube, then remember to take off the tourniquet before you pull out the needle. Then we would instruct the students to turn to their neighbor, and practice drawing blood. I loved the moment of terror in their eyes, and was always gratified to see that the terror of drawing blood was greater than the terror of blood being drawn.

Most of the time, they got it on the first stick. But sometimes, a student just couldn't get it. I would walk by and gently instruct them, and then, if they had tried a second time, I would offer up my veins. I have excellent veins—dark blue bulgy veins that show clearly through my skin. They are a medical student's dream, and many UTMB students drew their first vial of blood from me. During the orientation months, my bruised forearms were a badge of honor. Every awkward stick that I took was one spared a patient.

I RETURNED WITH a dermatologist volunteer, a kind but business-like older man, and did the biopsy. I shot half a cc of lidocaine into our patient's leg, and checked that it was numb. The blade, when I began to cut, was awkward. It took me longer than it would have for an experienced doctor. I couldn't get the blade angled under the last bit, so the piece of skin I'd cut off was dangling. I looked around for forceps, but they were still on the counter, sealed in autoclaved sterility. The doctor didn't offer them, so I grasped the dangling bit of skin with my gloved hand. I remembered our patient's hepatitis as the blade swiped perilously close to my finger. Biopsy done, I stopped the bleeding, and placed the sample in fluid to send it to the lab.

With the dermatologist in the room, our patient reverted to the usual calm mask of gratefulness. She sat quietly while I did the biopsy, then grasped my arm and said, "Thank you." The dermatologist never knew what had gone on.

It's painful to be told that the care my clinic gives is humiliating to patients. Even so, I'm glad that I'm not such an authority figure that the conversation can't even begin. Was she thanking me for doing the biopsy, or for hearing her out? Maybe she was thanking me for just getting that one thing done, so she could go home.

The next time I do a shave biopsy, I'll do it better. I'll begin with the forceps ready, and I'll be able to make one smooth cut. This is how medical training works: you count on your mentors to show you the way, and you learn as you go. You make mistakes as a student—more than residents make, and far more than fully qualified doctors make. Most of the time, your mistakes get caught by your superiors before you can do any real harm. But sometimes they don't get caught.

The problem, of course, is that these mistakes happen systematically, and not just to anyone. They happen to the uninsured and to people on Medicaid or county indigent programs. They happen to free-clinic patients, prisoners, and undocumented people. They happen to working-class whites and people of color.

If you are a patient at a private clinic—as I am myself—then you can be pretty sure that most of your doctor's mistakes have already been made. They were made on the bodies of the poor.

CHAPTER 21

WHEN I BECAME A STUDENT DIRECTOR, HTIN AUNG PASSED his keys off to me. Htin had been a great director, the most obsessive and dedicated of all the student directors, and he was going on to residency at the Mayo Clinic. "This is the key for the front door," he said. "This is the key to the chapel. This is the key to the medication closet in the hallway. This is the key to the counseling room." He went on and on, flipping through so many keys that I knew I would never remember them.

Becoming a student director at St. Vincent's meant that my duties changed. I was still a volunteer, but I was no longer primarily responsible for seeing patients (though directors would often see very complex patients who needed continuity of care). Instead, my job was to keep the clinic running.

There were ten directors, all of us in our last year of medical school, and we were all volunteers. We were responsible for staffing three clinics a week: Tuesday and Thursday nights, as well as Saturday mornings. Each clinic needed at least two directors, but ideally, four or more. We would also meet once a month on a Monday evening and, along with Dr. Beach, talk through any issues that had come up in clinic. Outside of those meetings and the actual clinics, we each had various responsibilities: coordinating volunteer sign-ups, making sure faculty doctors would be at the clinic, finding and organizing medication donations, fund-raising, representing the student-run clinic at St. Vincent's House meetings. There were also often small tasks to be done: a biopsy had been done but the doctor hadn't signed the form, for example, so a director would run to campus to track down the doctor. Somebody's medications had been mailed to the clinic but they had moved into a shelter in Houston, so the meds needed to be mailed to them. It went on and on.

The actual clinics were the heart of our work. On a typical Tuesday, I would show up to the clinic around four p.m. By then, our waiting room was usually full of patients and families waiting for their four thirty appointments. I'd walk in and say hello to the ladies working the reception desk, wave to patients I knew, and then head back to the banana room—the director's office, which had a painting of a banana on the door. (It was part of a healthy-foods themed mural that stretched around that part of the clinic.) I'd unlock the office and start setting up: logging on to computers, getting the safe open to remove prescription pads and the keys to the lab, setting out laptops for the volunteers to use. Often another director had beat me to the office and was catching up on paperwork. Somebody would check our box in the front office for new lab results, and start pulling charts to call patients back about their lab results.

Things would get briefly crazy around four fifteen when the volunteers all rolled in. We had eight exam rooms, plus two overflow rooms—the chapel and a counselor's office—where we could see patients. This meant that we could have ten teams, with a maximum of three students per team. The number of volunteers who actually showed up ebbed and flowed with school schedules. In August, the clinic would fill with brand-new med students eager to volunteer. On the night before a med-school test, we might pull in mostly physician assistant students. And over the holidays and summer we often struggled to get enough volunteers. We'd get on the St. Vincent's Facebook page and send out an SOS—*We need volunteers right now. There are* kolaches. Or *We need Spanish-speaking volunteers. There are sandwiches.* Or *We need upper-level students. There is pizza.* Keeping the food funded was a constant struggle, but it was important to show our volunteers that we appreciated them. Also, fed medical students are better, kinder medical students.

When Tay, our brilliant front-office manager, brought back the charts, we would break students into teams and send them out. Then, quiet would fall over the banana room, broken only by the murmur of a director making lab callbacks.

The quiet was brief, because before long our volunteers would start rocking up with questions. "How can I schedule this patient for an eye exam for his diabetes?" "Do we have any more of those giant Q-tips?" "Is there a counselor here tonight?" "My patient has a colostomy, but he can't afford colostomy bags. Can we get him colostomy bags?" (This question precipitates a brief bout of cursing the doctor or system that will do a multi-thousand-dollar surgery connecting a patient's colon to the wall of his abdomen, but won't provide him with plastic bags to catch his shit, then a furious discussion of whether we actually have colostomy bags and where they are, and why isn't his surgeon following him anyway?) "What do I do with this urine sample?" "Do we prescribe Klonopin?" "Can you look at this rash?" "This guy just had a stent put in his heart and they sent him here for follow-up, so what am I supposed to do with that?" "Do we give out glucometers?" "I think this X-ray report says this guy's back is broken." "Does anybody speak Spanish?"

The directors would field these questions, and welcome the doctors as they rolled in around five, and then the students would present their patients to us. We would coach them a little bit on how to present to the attending, bring up options for their differential diagnosis, and remind them to get the patient's height and weight. We would also field any emergent issues: If a patient had chest pain, we'd quickly make sure they didn't need to go to the ER. If somebody was bleeding, we'd supply gauze. If a biopsy was going to be done, we'd get the equipment. If somebody was about to have their lights turned off in their apartment, we'd refer them to the front desk for utilities assistance. If somebody had a child, we'd refer them to be evaluated for Medicaid eligibility. If a student was crying, we'd talk quietly with them. If somebody needed a medication they couldn't afford, we'd help the student start filling out the forms to apply for assistance. If somebody needed a chest X-ray, we'd look up the price, e-mail Dr. Beach to approve funding, and make a referral. If there was a patient in the waiting room who didn't have an appointment, one of us directors would triage them to figure out how urgently they needed to be seen.

After the student presented to us, we'd send him or her off to present to an attending doctor. The attending and the students would see the patient together, then come back to the banana room again so a director could give and document medication samples or donated meds, sign the chart, and schedule a follow-up appointment. The student would then head off to a laptop to finish writing the note on the patient, which we directors would also double check.

Practicing medicine as a student director at St. Vincent's meant having a fund of knowledge not just about disease and treatment, but also about the clinic itself, the social systems in our area, and the emotional experience of our volunteers. It meant keeping our patients and the clinic afloat, and trying to make sure our volunteers were supported through the intense experience of caring for struggling patients. So we directors just tried to do everything we could. We never knew enough, and relied on one another constantly. I became the person who knows about access to care; Julian understood ear, nose, and throat issues; Sarah was an expert in students' needs; Dave handled clinic finances; our junior director Jacqueline was great at doing pap smears. Once the questions started rolling in, they never stopped until the last patient had been seen.

Sometimes, the last patient would get out the door at seven thirty, but sometimes it was at nine thirty. When the last notes were in and the volunteers were gone, we would lock up the computers, shut the safe, turn off all the lights, and walk out front across the basketball court, past the community garden, and down the cracked sidewalk to our cars. One director would have snagged the vials of blood from the lab to drop off at the UTMB emergency room.

I always liked that task. I would drive Box up to the emergency room and park next to the ambulances, then head inside. If the labs were only blood samples, I'd put them in the pneumatic tube in the ER to send them to the lab. But if there were pap smears or urine samples, I'd walk through the silent labyrinth of the nighttime hospital, passing from one building to the next.

I liked glancing down the hallways and through the open doors of rooms as I went. Sometimes there would be a bright-lit tableau, almost like a diorama: two young men at a bedside, each holding the hand of an elderly woman whose face was turned away. A woman in maroon scrubs pushing a giant X-ray machine down a hallway. Two doctors quietly writing. The nighttime hospital felt calm and peaceful after an evening at St. Vincent's.

After dropping off the labs, I would drive back down the emergency room ramp and head to Arlan's, the local grocery store, to get a beer. Everybody shops at Arlan's, and a time or two I ran into patients whom I had just seen at the clinic. "Well, I reckon you need a beer, after all that," one woman said to me.

"Yes, ma'am," I said. Then I would go home and sit on the porch to have my beer. Sometimes my housemates would join me.

"Ah, your postclinic beer," Natasha would say.

"Indeed," I would say. "May they pry it from my cold, dead hands."

From the porch, we could see UTMB just across the street. The campus hummed and buzzed and glowed all night, with the giant laboratories blowing steam into the night air. Sometimes I would look at the hospital tower and wonder why my St. Vincent's patients couldn't just be let in. And sometimes there would be a breeze blowing across the island from the Gulf, and I would just lean back and let the evening fall away from me.

CHAPTER 22

MALACHAI CAME TO GALVESTON FROM OUT OF STATE, AND he could not or would not explain how he got here. He walked into the clinic one day, told the student who saw him he was worried about a bump on his head, and asked to go off of his schizophrenia medication. Also, he asked for a testicle exam. He said there was nothing wrong with his testicles; he just wanted an exam. The bump on his head was a benign mole, and his schizophrenia, if he really had it, was well controlled. The student was a second-year, and she emerged from the encounter feeling thoroughly flustered. "Am I supposed to do a testicle exam?" she asked me.

"Um," I said, "a testicle exam isn't really indicated unless there's something wrong. Pain, or a lump, or something. Let's talk to an attending."

So then the attending got involved, and he also could not piece together Malachai's story, nor did he think a testicle exam was warranted. The encounter struck him as strange enough that he decided to Google Malachai, and what he found was so troubling that he came into the banana room saying, "We can't see this patient. He can't be seen by students. He needs to go somewhere else."

I was in the banana room with Sarah, another director. Sarah looked up from her computer and pointed out the obvious: "I'm not sure that's an option," she said. "If he's uninsured, there's not really anywhere to send him."

"No, this is serious," the attending said. "This guy has a serious criminal record. I don't think he should be here."

"But, a lot of our patients have criminal records," I said. I remembered what I had told a junior student just the week before:

> Prison is just a place where they send poor people and black people. So if your patient has been in prison, you want to be alert for the possibility of posttraumatic stress disorder, because prison can cause it and because having it in the first place is a risk factor for going to prison. You should also think of certain infectious diseases that are prevalent among prisoners: tuberculosis, hepatitis C, HIV. You do not need to worry about what they supposedly did. If they're here, they're your patient.

Given the rate of incarceration of African Americans, a free clinic housed in a historically African American community center in Texas could not exactly be turning people away because they had criminal records. It would be against the spirit of the House.

But the attending wouldn't budge, and it seemed that the request for a testicle exam was the kicker, along with whatever the attending had discovered through his Google search. "This guy is obviously dangerous," he said. "He could be on the lam. He should not be seen by students."

Sarah's face wrinkled up, and I felt my own eyebrows raise. We were not eager to tell any patient that they could not be seen here; to do so was, essentially, to say they would not get medical care at all. The situation was not fair, but it was very clear.

Sarah and I reached a compromise with the attending: we would reschedule Malachai for psychiatry night, so he could get his schizophrenia care in order, and make him "directors only." Sarah and I would see him together (because the attending insisted that no woman see him alone).

So, Sarah and I went in to introduce ourselves. Malachai had a gentle demeanor; he nodded slowly along as we spoke and agreed to come back to the clinic on Thursday, for psychiatry night.

"Can I stop taking these pills now, please?" he asked.

"Keep taking them for now," Sarah said. "Let's not make any changes until you get a chance to meet with our psychiatry doctors."

Malachai nodded, and we all shook hands. Sarah and I stood, but he remained sitting.

"Is there something else you need?" Sarah asked.

"Yes," he said. "I would like to learn how to make more friends."

"Oh," Sarah said gently. "That's a good thing to learn about. We'll talk about that on Thursday."

"Oh, okay," he said. "Thank you." Then he stood and we showed him to the front door.

The sign in the waiting room at St. Vincent's says, ALL ARE WEL-COME HERE. For a long time, I took pride in volunteering at a clinic where all patients were truly welcome. But eventually I realized that I, too, felt welcome here. It was my House. And so the fact that a volunteer doctor wanted to ban a patient because of his criminal record troubled me. I decided to take the issue to Mr. Jackson.

IF ASKED TO DESCRIBE HIMSELF, Mr. Michael Thomas Jackson will say that he is first a child of God, and then a male of the species, and then a man of African descent. He is also an Episcopal lay minister, and was the director of St. Vincent's House during my years there. He takes the welcoming nature of St. Vincent's very seriously. "You are not just welcome here. You are *expected* here," he says. "The next person walking through that front door could be Christ Christself." Mr. Jackson does not ascribe gender to the Lord.

Like me, Mr. Jackson also came through that door in his own unique way. He grew up in Washington, D.C., the son of a police officer and a CIA worker. His mother trained all her supervisors at the CIA but never got promoted; his father kept failing the D.C.

sergeant's test by a couple of points. Once upon a time his mother's family was Roman Catholic in South Carolina, but then they were told they would have to sit in the balcony at church. Mr. Jackson's grandmother said, "Well, that's not going to work," so they became Episcopalians. His mother's family was eventually run out of South Carolina because the patriarch was organizing people for black voting rights, and so the family moved to the District.

Mr. Jackson started school in 1954, in the first year of desegregation. His first political activity was in ninth grade, and it involved lobbying Congress for better books in the public schools. (The D.C. school budget is controlled by Congress.) The racial mix of his schools changed with the times and with his family's financial circumstance. He started out in a high school that was 60 percent black, but white flight happened so fast in the sixties that by the time he graduated it was 99 percent. He decided not to include a picture of himself when he applied to college, and he was accepted to Rutgers. His close circle of friends went to all the top colleges: Columbia, Penn, Harvard, Yale. It felt for a moment like things were changing.

But Rutgers was turbulent in 1968: classes got shut down for bomb scares, and the war was on. Mr. Jackson was not a formal member of the Black Panther Party, but many of his friends were, and the party was influential in leading him to a life of service. At that time, the Panthers were working to feed the people and running free medical clinics, but were also supporting armed revolution.* "I was a militant," Mr. Jackson says, "for a time."

But then, he says, love saved him. He fell in love with a woman, who introduced him to circles of people who were learning about nonviolence. He became convinced that armed revolution was not going to work in America. "Most of our models for revolution were taken from the developing world," he says. "Ché was big. But armed

---

* For more on the Black Panthers and medical care, see Alondra Nelson, *Body and Soul: The Black Panther Party and the Fight against Medical Discrimination* (Minneapolis: University of Minnesota Press, 2011).

revolt was not going to be the way this place was going to change. We couldn't outgun the police or the military."

Even so, Mr. Jackson does not believe that the Black Panthers were so violently repressed by the state because they were advocating armed revolution. Rather, it was because they built bridges with other communities: "The Panthers had to go because they were coalition builders," he says. "They built coalitions with other communities. Malcolm had to go. Anytime you step out of segregation activities to unifying activities, you will be eliminated."

Mr. Jackson committed himself to working to better the world, and to doing it as nonviolently as possible. He married in 1974, and then felt his first tugs toward the ministry. But it was not for a few more years, after separating from his then-wife and spending a year in Jamaica, that he was ready to tell the bishop that he could commit his life to Christ. And so it happened, though he did not finish divinity school. He was homeless for a minute, then became a lay minister. He wanted to be a prison chaplain, but he was called—literally called on the phone, by the bishop—to Galveston.

"I knew nothing about St. Vincent's and I got lost every time I tried to get here," he says. Galveston felt like being sent back to the hood. But they interviewed him at a restaurant on the seawall, and he'd always wanted to live near the ocean.

"I'm a radical heretic," he tells me. "God is love."

MR. JACKSON'S OFFICE is behind the reception area at St. Vincent's House. When you walk into the House, you hit the waiting room first. The hallway to your right leads to the clinic, and the hallway to the left leads to the food bank, the chapel, and the offices. So on the morning I decided to track Mr. Jackson down to talk about Malachai, he was in his office fielding phone calls but he smiled and waved me in. I took a seat among the bookshelves and toys and sculptures, next to a giant stuffed banana with dreadlocks and a Jamaican-flag-colored hat, across the desk from Mr. Jackson. The nameplate on his desk said, "Servant in Chief." He passed me a little metal brain teaser to play with while he finished on the phone.

"Rachel!" he said after hanging up, smiling broadly. "What brings you in here on this beautiful Monday when there is no clinic?"

"Hi, Mr. Jackson," I said, smiling. "I wanted to talk with you about a patient." And so I explained about Malachai: the request for a testicle exam, the Google search, the attending's fear. How we figured out a way not to turn him away, but I was struggling with the notion that the student clinic might be out of step with the welcoming philosophy of the House.

Mr. Jackson listened and nodded. He already knew Malachai: he knew Malachai was working on his GED at the St. Vincent's school, that he didn't have family to rely on, that he was trading day labor for room and board at a safe house on the island.

"Listen, Rachel," he said. "Every patient is a miracle. Malachai coming through that door at all—that was a miracle."

"Well, yeah," I said. "Okay. But then we shouldn't be banning him!"

"He's not banned," he said. "He may not be able to work with that one doctor, but he's still welcome here."

"But what if he needs to see a regular internal medicine doctor?"

"Well, you may not be able to get him everything he needs," Mr. Jackson said. And then he gave me a history lesson. He talked about the years when the student-run clinic was just once a week, and never in the summers, how it expanded gradually. "I worked for years for us *not* to be a health home," he said. He had envisioned the student-run clinic as a portal to care, where people would come to get triaged and then sent on to a higher level of consistent care. But the higher level fell through.

"You all," he said, "can't always give your patients everything they need. You can't. But one is better than zero."

"One is better than zero?" I asked.

"Sure. Okay. So you have this patient, and he comes in at zero: no doctor, no medications, nothing. And you want to get him up to five, don't you?"

"Yes."

"But you can't get him to five, because five takes, say, an operating room. But you can get him to one. Even just coming through this door, that's getting to one. And one is better than zero."

Over the course of the year, I would have this conversation with Mr. Jackson many times. He always said that one is better than zero, and I always said that one is still an injustice when somebody needs five. We were both right. And eventually I learned that Mr. Jackson's relative comfort with patients being at one rather than five was related to his belief that medical interventions are neither necessarily good nor essential to healing. For him, the heart of medical care is not in medications or surgeries: it is in one human being recognizing another human being, who is suffering. The heart of medicine is exactly the thing we do well at St. Vincent's, even when we can't do all the rest. Although he himself is insured, Mr. Jackson gets his annual physical at the student-run free clinic.

Over time, I have come closer to believing what Mr. Jackson believes. But I still argue that the trappings of medicine—the surgeries, the chemotherapy, the interventions—not only sometimes do fix what ails us but also are important symbols of the pledge that a person's life matters. As technical and cold as medical interventions can be, they are often society's best way of proving that a person's life does matter.

Mr. Jackson told me that we doctors are just instruments. We start off as technicians, he said, thinking we know everything. We become physicians when we are honest about our mistakes, and start listening a little harder. After a while, he said, "You transcend into healing. You realize that you are a medium for the whole process. It isn't you."

MALACHAI CAME BACK on Thursday's psychiatry night, and the visit was totally uneventful. He would stay on his medication, and would apply for assistance from a pharmaceutical company to pay for it. I walked through the paperwork with him, and he had no recent pay stubs or tax returns, so we sent a letter off to the IRS requesting proof that he did not file taxes. When that came back, we would see about getting him the medication. In the meantime, we gave him a month's worth of meds from our stock, and made him an appointment to see us again.

"Can we be friends?" Malachai asked the psychiatrist.

The psychiatrist smiled. "Of course we can," he said, shaking Malachai's hand. "We are friends, and I'll see you here in clinic."

After we left the room, the psychiatrist turned to Sarah and me. "I think he has some cognitive disability," he said. "Maybe mild mental retardation."

Sarah and I went back to the office, and I told her about my talk with Mr. Jackson. Malachai will still be supported by the House, even if he can't come to Tuesday clinics. We both felt relieved, but a little puzzled and a little angry over what had happened on Tuesday.

"He seems like a completely gentle person to me," Sarah said, and I agreed.

WHEN WE TRAIN in Hospital Galveston, the prison hospital, our mentors advise us not to look up our patients' criminal records. To do say may change our ability to care for our patients in ways that we cannot predict. When in the prison hospital, I never cared to look up anyone's record. I figured I was above it, anyway: I knew that the prison system was racist and rigged. I wouldn't judge anybody for having committed a crime.

But I could not stop wondering what had frightened that attending doctor at St. Vincent's so much—especially when Malachai came off as a perfectly gentle human being, whose story didn't make sense because he had a cognitive disability. So one night, my curiosity got the better of me, and I Googled him.

I wish I had not done it.

The story that came up was bizarre. Malachai hadn't hurt any people, exactly, but he'd been arrested for stalking a woman in a very frightening way. There was a picture of him in custody, looking wild-eyed and confused.

This was difficult to square with the quiet man I'd met, who painstakingly wrote his name in all capital letters on the IRS form. I discussed it with Sarah, who confessed that she, too, looked him up. To do so is not illegal or strictly unethical, but we both felt that it was unwise.

We went on seeing Malachai, who became a regular and beloved face around the House on psychiatry nights. One night he said that he would rather live somewhere else, because the man he was living with didn't pay him for his work. We talked to him about looking for jobs in the newspaper, but we kept in mind Mr. Jackson's sense that the living arrangement was a good one for Malachai. He could easily fall off the edge of society, beyond which there is no safety net. *One is better than zero*, I reminded myself, when the IRS rejected our application for proof of nonfiling and we gave Malachai another month's worth of sample drugs.

One night Malachai asked me if we could be friends, and I gently said no. "I will be your medical student," I said, "and I will do my best to care for you in this clinic." But that was all.

CHAPTER 23

JACOB CAME INTO THE DIRECTOR'S OFFICE WITH A CHART
in his hands, looking shaken. "Can I present to you?" he asked.

"Sure," I said. "Give me one sec." I finished the note I was writing
in a patient's electronic medical record—labs suggest that rheumatoid
arthritis is not adequately controlled on current regimen, consistent
with symptoms, follow-up scheduled in one month—and turned to
Jacob. "Go ahead."

"Okay. So. This is Ms. Blair. She's a thirty-nine-year-old African
American woman with an abdominal mass, who presents today with
a CT scan suggesting cancer."

"Whoa," I said.

"Yeah," Jacob said.

"You have the CT?"

"I have the printout they gave her," Jacob explained. "It was at a
hospital on the mainland. She's had this mass in her belly for three
years now, and it's growing. It's like the size of a football. But she
doesn't have insurance, obviously, because she's here. Anyway, we
saw her here last month for carpal tunnel syndrome, but also on exam
she had this big mass. So we advised her to go to the ER and maybe
get imaging. They did a CT in the emergency room, and then they
sent her back here."

Jacob handed me the printout. The radiologist who had analyzed her CT wrote that it looked like the mass was growing into her intestines. "A large mesenteric mass of solid and cystic components, possible uterine or ovarian origin . . . suspicious for sarcoma, carcinoma . . ."—in short, cancer. Possibly.

"So did they do a biopsy?" I asked. You can't actually diagnose cancer from an imaging study; you have to do a biopsy to get a sample of the tissue.

"No," Jacob said. "They just did the CT, and told her to come here."

"Okay," I said, feeling annoyed with the hospital. "So they decided their potential cancer patient should come to the student-run free clinic. Great idea."

Jacob shrugged.

"Any other symptoms?" I asked.

"Some burning after she eats, and belly pain. But nothing else."

"No weight loss?" I asked.

"No weight loss."

"And on physical exam?"

"Well," Jacob said, "the mass is in her lower abdomen, and it's really obvious. You can see it. It looks like she's pregnant. And when you feel, it's hard and basically smooth. Nontender. Nonmobile. But, listen, I . . ."

"You?" I said gently. It was strange to see Jacob so shaken. He was just a second-year student, but he was an experienced volunteer who came to almost every clinic day at St. Vincent's. On Saturday mornings, he would wake up at seven to go to the Luke Society homeless clinic, held in a parking lot downtown, and then come to St. Vincent's at ten. He had cared for cancer patients, and always seemed unflappable: calm, smiling, concrete. When things went badly with a patient, he would go home and read a book with dragons in it. I trust him.

"The thing is," Jacob said quickly, "I think I just told her that she has cancer."

"Oh, my gosh," I said.

"You know, by accident. She had been to the ER, and they did this CT so I thought they explained it to her. But she didn't know."

"What happened?" I asked.

"Well, I said, 'So they told you that you might have cancer?' and she just looked at me and shook her head," Jacob said. "I am so sorry. I just didn't think about it. I'm so sorry."

"Oh, Jacob," I said. "It's not your fault. The hospital never should have put you in that situation." I was trying to be gentle and focus on Jacob, but my annoyance flared again. How could the hospital be so irresponsible, sending this patient to us without telling her the results of the CT? Did they really think it was right to off-load that duty onto students? Jacob was just a second-year med student.

Then again, maybe I was at fault. I was one of the directors of this clinic, and I had let a junior student walk into this situation on his own. A senior student would know to begin by asking the patient what she understood about the CT. If the patient didn't say the word "cancer," a senior student would know to bring an attending in. All of us directors trusted Jacob's skills so much that we always asked him to see patients on his own when we were short on volunteers. But maybe I had let him down by not making sure that he had adequate support.

Jacob was still standing there, his shoulders slumped. "I just didn't think," he said softly.

"Jacob," I said again. "You didn't do anything wrong. Let's get Dr. Black, and let's figure out what to do."

"Burnout," Susan McCammon once said, "is not in the Jacob Lin mentality." Jacob comes from the Houston suburbs, and he went to a smaller college where he double majored in biology and chemistry. He also volunteered one hundred hours per semester as part of a service fraternity. His favorite service activity was called Agape Meal, where volunteers would sit down and eat with homeless people. There, Jacob learned that homelessness was, as he calls it, "just a situation." Some people are homeless for decades, but for some, it was a temporary state—jobs fell through, apartments kicked families out, and they were on the streets.

When he came to Galveston and started medical school, Jacob was amazed at the amount of free time he suddenly had. *What am I going to do with all this free time?* he wondered. Within two weeks of starting school, he began volunteering at St. Vincent's.

The first night Jacob came, it was ob-gyn night, and he couldn't volunteer because he hadn't been trained to do speculum exams. He came back the next Tuesday, on dermatology night, and his very first patient had delusions of parasitosis—that is, the patient experienced the sensation of bugs crawling on her skin, but there was no dermatological cause of that experience. Jacob says that the patient got really angry when the dermatologist explained this to her.

"But everyone else was so nice!" he said. "The doctor, and the student directors. They were all really great. Everybody was really nice. Except for the patient. She yelled at us. But anyway, I loved it."

So Jacob felt comfortable at St. Vincent's early on, and with the copious free time of a first-year medical student who has never had to struggle for a grade in his life, Jacob began coming to St. Vincent's two or three times a week. Just as I had, he learned how to practice medicine there.

The first few months were a honeymoon. "At that time, I was still under the impression that there was a safety net," he said. "I didn't realize that we were the safety net."

THE HONEYMOON ENDED with Jacob's first cancer patient. Lex Klein was sixty-one and living in the Salvation Army shelter in Galveston. He'd had pain in his throat for a year, and had been to the emergency room twice: once, a doctor prescribed him penicillin. It didn't help. The next time he went to the ER, they did a CT scan and found a tumor at the base of his tongue. But he couldn't get medical care—he wasn't old enough to qualify for Medicare, and as an adult man with no dependent children, he was ineligible for Medicaid in Texas. He started taking handfuls of ibuprofen to try to dull the pain.

So one night, Mr. Klein rode his bicycle to St. Vincent's, and the student directors called Susan McCammon—who by then had become our regular ENT consultant—to come and meet him. She brought the equipment to do a biopsy into the clinic, and Dr. Schnadig, a UTMB pathologist, read the biopsy results for free. It was cancer.

Jacob was at one of Mr. Klein's first appointments, and he kind of adopted him. Along with Julian, a student director who was planning to go into ENT, Jacob started seeing him every Tuesday evening.

At the time, St. Vincent's had a blanket policy of not prescribing opiates—drugs that are not only addictive but can also be sold on the street. Established clinics have solid ways of monitoring the use of these drugs—regular urine drug screens, for example, to make sure that the person prescribed the medications is actually taking them. As a student-run clinic, we couldn't even guarantee that our patients would always be seen by the same provider, and we worried that pre-scribing these drugs might do more harm than good.

In my graduate courses, however, I was learning that this policy was problematic. Poor people are very likely to be denied access to opiates—which, as imperfect as they are, are the indicated medica-tion for cancer pain. Pharmacies in poor neighborhoods often don't stock opiates, so it can be hard to get the drugs even if you have a prescription. And African Americans in general are very likely to be untreated or undertreated for pain. Although studies show that Afri-can Americans are less likely than whites to abuse opiates, doctors seem to profile black patients as addicts or potential addicts, and fail to prescribe the appropriate drugs.

We had good reasons not to prescribe opiates at St. Vincent's, but we were also part of a bigger problem: as a safety-net clinic housed in a historically African American community center, we were a classic example of why black patients' pain went undertreated.

So along came Mr. Klein, with his incredibly painful cancer growing in his throat, and we knew it had been there for a year and that he still wasn't getting chemotherapy for it. Even with treatment, throat cancer kills 50 percent of people. And, ideally, patients should go from diagnosis to treatment in less than one hundred days.

After the biopsy, Jacob and Dr. McCammon came into the student director's office. "I need a prescription pad for a triplicate," Dr. McCammon said.

"Um," I said, "I'm not sure we have that. What's a triplicate?"

"I need to write for methadone for Mr. Klein. For his pain. And it's a controlled substance, so it goes on a special prescription pad."

"Oh," I said. The office was full of students; someone was on the phone, and two students were rifling through the sample medications on the shelf. It was noisy. "Yeah. We don't have that."

"So, how do you prescribe opiates?" Susan asked.

"Um," I said, feeling embarrassed, "we don't prescribe them."

"He has cancer," she said, looking at me flatly and speaking slowly, as if I were a dim specimen of a medical student. "Pain control with opiates is part of the standard of care."

"I'm with you," I said. "I want his pain to be treated. But we don't prescribe them here."

Dr. McCammon did the sensible thing, and brought her own prescription pad to write a prescription for methadone for Mr. Klein. So our policy changed a bit: with cancer patients, we would do our best to handle prescribing opiates. But it turned out not to be as simple as that. Mr. Klein had managed to get access to a little bit of money, through a bank account set up by his brother, for the medication. He had a debit card. So he would ride his bicycle to the pharmacy and try to use the debit card for the methadone, but the debit card had someone else's name on it. Sometimes he would get turned away. Dr. McCammon took to meeting him at the pharmacy so she could stand there and tell the pharmacist that yes, this was her patient, and yes, he needed methadone. But even then it was complicated: one week, a pharmacy would have methadone, and the next week it wouldn't. Mr. Klein would end up bicycling all over the island trying to get his medication. And that wasn't so easy because, on top of the bicycling and the hassle and having to get back to the Salvation Army every night in time to be let in before curfew, he also had cancer.

"It was dangerous for him to have the methadone," Jacob explained. "It could have gotten stolen. I don't know what would have happened to him if other people had found out he had methadone. But somehow he managed to keep it secret."

Pain control, of course, was not all that Jacob wanted to offer Mr. Klein. He also wanted to get him the chemotherapy, surgery, and radiation that he needed. And so he set about trying, with a kind of dogged diligence that I have never seen in anyone else. He worked with Susan to amass the paperwork to apply for care for Mr. Klein through the UTMB Casebook system, and then sat quietly while Susan told him that he had been denied. He called around to all the local hospitals. He found out that the American Cancer Society would provide transportation to appointments for Mr. Klein, and so then he started calling hospitals in Houston. He helped him get together an application for the Galveston County indigent care program. None of it worked.

All this time, Mr. Klein kept feeling hopeful. He really believed that Jacob and the others at St. Vincent's were going to get him treatment. As the rejections rolled in, he would accept the news calmly. "He had tremendous faith in all of us," Jacob said, "that we were going to be able to help him."

Jacob didn't know how to feel about that faith. He didn't think he deserved it. After a long time, he no longer felt hopeful that Mr. Klein was going to get treatment. He no longer believed that the medical system was working, or that people who truly needed help could get it. He would hang up the phone after another frustrating call, weeping with anger. He started blasting Nine Inch Nails in his apartment. "Nine Inch Nails helped a lot, actually," he said.

Susan counseled Jacob on hope. "I learned that there are a lot of different things you can hope for," Jacob said, when hoping to live no longer feels like an option. You can hope for a death that feels like part of life, that is more pain-free and gentle than you ever expected. You can hope for forgiveness, or reconciliation—with family, with God. You can hope for a good life in the time you have. Gently, in the clinic room at St. Vincent's, Susan taught Jacob how to talk about these kinds of hope with Mr. Klein.

Early in medical school, Jacob never expected that he would be having conversations about hope. "I'm more of a concrete person," he said. He is fluent in the immune effects of hyperglycemia, the morphology of *Giardia*, the pharmacology of beta-blockers. "I can get touchy-feely when the situation arises," he said. "And it arose, so I did that. But no, I never expected to be in that situation."

Then in May, a full eight months after Mr. Klein first showed up at St. Vincent's, he was accepted into the Galveston County indigent care system. So hope, the old-fashioned kind of hope for survival, swelled again.

The county said that Mr. Klein would need to live in walking distance of the hospital if he didn't have a car. But the hospital was on the mainland, and Mr. Klein was still living in the Salvation Army shelter. His brother came through and bought him a trailer near the hospital. And things began to happen.

After moving to the mainland, Mr. Klein would call Jacob every two weeks or so to update him. He was scheduled to begin chemo-therapy in July. He had scans done to look for the spread of cancer around his body. He even went into surgery, where they placed a feeding tube in his stomach to prepare him for the removal of the throat cancer. He would be unable to eat by mouth for quite a while.

But the throat cancer was never removed. Because, in a final ago-nizing turn, the county said in July that Mr. Klein no longer qualified for indigent care because he owned the trailer. He was too wealthy.

Mr. Klein kept calling Jacob for a while, once a month or so. After a time, the calls stopped. Jacob still has the number in his phone, but he doesn't want to call it. Some part of him just doesn't want to know.

JACOB SAYS NOW THAT his experience with Mr. Klein helped prepare him to care for Vicki Blair, the woman with the large mass in her belly.

Together, Jacob and I talked with Dr. Black, who volunteers at St. Vincent's every Tuesday. She is a no-nonsense doctor with impeccable credentials and a great bedside manner. I knew she would be the right person to help Ms. Blair.

The three of us knocked and entered Ms. Blair's room, and sat down around her. She was sitting in a chair with her back to the wall, dressed in athletic pants and a T-shirt. Dr. Black introduced herself and me, and then said, "I understand you got this CT scan done at Shoreline. And that Jacob told you that the doctors there thought that it might look like cancer." I felt Jacob tense up beside me.

Ms. Blair nodded.

"I am sorry," Dr. Black said. "I know that's not good news, and it can be really scary."

Ms. Blair nodded again.

"I want you to understand, though, that we don't yet know if it is cancer. There's obviously something going on, but a CT scan doesn't diagnose it."

"Well, what do you think it is then?" Ms. Blair asked.

"I don't know," Dr. Black said. "It could be cancer. But it could also be a kind of growth that isn't cancer, or isn't dangerous."

"So are y'all going to figure that out?" Ms. Blair asked. Her eyebrows were raised, and she looked skeptical. Which was right, I figured, because she had already gotten the runaround from a hospital. Why would she think that a free clinic could help her?

"We're going to try," Dr. Black said. "We need to do a biopsy, where we take a needle and look at a sample of the tissue inside you. So our next step is going to be figuring out how to get you that biopsy."

"Figuring it out?" Ms. Blair asked.

Dr. Black nodded. I knew why she was hesitating to just say yes, we would do it. A lot of things had been done at St. Vincent's that don't happen in most primary care clinics—things like Mr. Klein's throat biopsy—but this would be a new one for us. We had never tried to do a biopsy through the wall of someone's abdomen. And I wasn't confident that we could do it, or should. What if there was a complication? What if she bled? I knew that in a worst-case scenario we could send her to UTMB in an ambulance. But was it safe to try this at all, with the nearest operating room at least fifteen minutes away? I could imagine the look on a surgeon's face, receiving a patient transported from St. Vincent's by ambulance and asking, "What the hell are they doing over there?" I could imagine a UTMB administrator calculating the cost of treating Ms. Blair for complications caused by a biopsy at St. Vincent's, and then picking up a telephone to start a cascade of decisions that would shut down the clinic. I could imagine our patients, then, having nowhere at all to go.

Then I looked at Ms. Blair. She was only ten years older than me. She was a mother. She was loved in the world, and she was struggling to trust us. Getting her the biopsy she needed might be a step toward earning her trust, showing her that somebody in the world of medicine believes that her life matters. But if something went wrong . . .

I looked around the room, from face to face. There was skeptical Vicki Blair with something growing in her belly, calm Dr. Black, and Jacob looking nervous but determined. And there I was, the person trying to keep this operation afloat.

Nothing about this was going to be easy, or simple. We were in over our heads.

CHAPTER 24

AT THE END OF CLINIC, WE HUDDLED AROUND DR. BLACK—
Jacob, a junior director named Jacqueline, two other doctors who
were volunteering that night, and me. In a clinic without social
workers, care coordination happened like this: Jacob suggested con-
tacting the ob-gyn doctors to make a Casebook application. I printed
out the forms for Ms. Blair to apply to the county indigent care program, and Jacqueline said maybe we could start with an endometrial
biopsy—but we ruled that plan out because our patient was already
having heavy bleeding and an endometrial biopsy could be risky.
Dr. Black called a pathologist, while another student director looked
at the CD Ms. Blair had brought to see whether we could see the
images of her CT scan.

"The pathologist would need to see the images," Dr. Black said,
"to know if it might be safe to do the biopsy in clinic." In all likeli-
hood, this biopsy would need to be guided by ultrasound.

"I'm worried," I told Dr. Black. "If something goes wrong with
this, what do we do?"

"We'll talk to the experts," Dr. Black said. "We won't do this if it
isn't safe."

As the preparations went forward, some part of my mind still hes-
itated to think this was a great idea. Other students were excited,

proud of the possibility that our little clinic might be able to offer such high-tech care. As much as we students wish the best for our patients, we also take some pride in caring for people with complex conditions—exactly the kind of patients who need more than we can really offer.

And so it happened. A month later, I stood in the doorway of a clinic room while Dr. Black and an interventional radiologist prepared to do the biopsy. A pathologist was also standing by. The radiologist had seen the images, and decided that she could safely guide a small needle through Ms. Blair's abdominal wall into the mass. With all the equipment in there—the ultrasound, the microscope, the bevy of white coats—our clinic room suddenly looked like an operating room. I felt a surge of pride. But then, as Ms. Blair came down the hall to the room with her face as calm and impassive as ever, I thought, *Oh my god. What are we doing here?*

Jacqueline and Jacob assisted on the biopsy, and were there a week later to give Ms. Blair her results: The biopsy had shown abnormal cells, consistent with a cancer of the uterus. She needed to get the mass removed. So she had hit the St. Vincent's wall: we were able to diagnose her with cancer, but unable to offer her the surgery she needed.

Some providers believe that the St. Vincent's wall is not one we should even approach: Why diagnose people if we can't make sure they will get treatment? It's too hard on the students, and not necessarily a great service to the patients. Susan McCammon believes otherwise: Sometimes doors open after a cancer diagnosis. Knowledge can be power; knowledge can be among the faint threads of support—like nonabandonment—that we offer to our unfunded patients.

Ms. Blair took the news, Jacqueline said, stoically. Jacqueline gave Ms. Blair her phone number, and made her a weekly standing appointment at St. Vincent's. This was beginning to be our cancer care routine: for patients with diagnosed cancers, we guarded weekly Tuesday appointments to make sure they could see the same providers and get any symptoms managed quickly as they emerged.

In these weekly appointments, Jacqueline began working with Ms.

Blair on putting together an application for insurance through the Affordable Care Act health exchange. Through her two part-time jobs, Ms. Blair made just barely enough money to qualify for subsidized insurance. But she was scraping by, and was not sure she could cover the cost of insurance even with a subsidy. Jacqueline counseled her to look for a plan that would cover a high percentage of the cost of care. Jacqueline walked her through the terminology that she was encountering on the insurance exchange, learning alongside her. Ms. Blair called on her own best resource: her supportive family, who pooled enough money to get her the insurance. When it finally came through, a few months after the biopsy at St. Vincent's, she immediately made an appointment at UTMB.

Jacqueline never felt a breakthrough with Ms. Blair. She never felt that trust developed, or that they became close. Ms. Blair cried only once. Jacqueline screened her for depression, but she wasn't depressed. She was just sad.

The doctors who did the surgery updated us on the results. The mass was removed completely, but it wasn't cancer. It was just a large growth in the uterus. And it undoubtedly needed to go, but it never would've threatened Ms. Blair's life. Jacqueline puzzled back through the studies—the CT, the biopsy—to try to figure out what had happened, why our diagnosis was wrong. A pathologist said that maybe the biopsy needle just happened to hit a pocket of abnormal cells.

So Jacqueline was left wondering if the whole thing had been worth it: the months of worry, telling a woman that she had cancer, and the effort that Ms. Blair's family had to make to pay for her insurance. After the surgery, Ms. Blair never again contacted St. Vincent's, Jacqueline, or Jacob.

One day, Jacqueline came up to me in the library on campus, and asked if we could talk.

"For sure," I said. We went out to a sunny bench outside the library. We could see nurses and medical students having lunch behind the hospital, and junior students rushing back and forth with their backpacks. The big clock next to us was still stuck at the time that Hurricane Ike had flooded through the campus five years before. Almost as soon as Jacqueline started talking, she began to cry. It was about Ms. Blair.

"I gave her my phone number," she said, "and I really want to call her, but I don't know if that's okay."

"Just to call her to check in on her?" I asked.

"Yeah." Jacqueline knew that the surgery had been successful, and that Ms. Blair wouldn't need further treatment, but she had no way of knowing if Ms. Blair herself was okay. And did she think it had been worth it, after all?

Students never entirely know what boundaries we are crossing in caring for patients at St. Vincent's. The fact of giving out your phone number could mean that boundaries were being violated—the fragile lines that, in some cases, help us medical providers keep some notion of having "normal lives."

On the other hand, I had given my number to a couple of patients, and I knew that the doctors I admired most—Dr. Beach and Dr. McCammon—had done the same. Jacqueline was afraid of turning into Dr. Beach, so exquisitely dedicated to his patients that he seemed unable to pull away from the medical school, from St. Vincent's, from us students. And yet she also knew she would, someday, become a doctor like that.

"Well, sure, I think that's okay," I said. "That's good medicine."

ONE DAY, JACQUELINE went in to do a pap smear on a patient whom two second-year students were seeing. When Jacqueline inserted the speculum and the woman's cervix popped into view, there was a bloody growth dangling from it. Jacqueline closed her eyes for one moment and reopened them: the growth was still there. It was as if Jacqueline could see already the months that lay ahead, the pain, the fear. The woman was alive and dying in that moment, rushing more quickly toward some precipice that, for this silent moment, only Jacqueline knew was there.

The woman's name was Gloria, and she had come in because she was postmenopausal, but had started bleeding. Jacqueline removed the speculum, apologized briefly to Gloria, and went to get the doctor.

Later, Jacqueline would wonder why she gave her phone number to Gloria, why she drove Gloria into Houston for an appointment at MD Anderson, why Gloria became the patient she worried over so much. Why this one, and not them all?

"I guess it's because she reminds me of my grandmother," Jacqueline said. Then she corrected herself. "I mean, my nanny." Gloria would ask after Jacqueline's family, call her tender nicknames in Spanish. "She thinks I'm the best," Jacqueline said, "even though we've had these really difficult encounters. I've felt like I was failing her from very early on, and through all that she calls me *cielo* and *princesa*."

JACQUELINE WAS RAISED in South Texas, and Gloria was raised in El Salvador.

Jacqueline's grandparents emigrated from Cuba, and hers was a family of doctors. Her father's father was an ophthalmologist in Cuba, then repeated residency in Detroit to become an American general practitioner. Jacqueline's own father became an oncologist. Her mother once refused to move to Port Arthur because "it smells." Jacqueline had a nanny, whom she loved. There is a Catholic shrine in the entryway to their house, and Jacqueline's mother often tells her to pray. Her father says that she will need God as a physician. Once you stop living in the world of black and white, and live all the time in the gray areas, he has told her, you need God.

Gloria had a husband and a chauffeur in El Salvador. But after she and her husband both lost their jobs, Gloria promised a coyote three thousand dollars to bring her north. She worked for a while in a shrimp factory in Virginia, saving enough money to pay off the coyote and to bring her daughter north. The daughter married an American citizen and doesn't involve herself much with Gloria, certainly not enough to help pay for Gloria's sons, her brothers, to come north. As for Gloria's husband, well, *Quien sabe?* So Gloria moved to Galveston, to live with a nephew and work in a hotel kitchen. She wore high yellow gloves that made the skin of her hands crack. And one day she arrived at St. Vincent's, and Jacqueline met her.

THE BLOODY GROWTH in Gloria's vagina was cancer. It was cervical cancer, which is generally among the better cancers to be diagnosed with at St. Vincent's. A federal law called the Breast and Cervical Cancer Prevention and Treatment Act of 2000 guarantees funding for both screening and treatment for these cancers to women living at or below 250 percent of the federal poverty level. This means that St. Vincent's patients can get mammograms for free, and when one of our pap smears is abnormal, we can refer the patient for treatment. Unfortunately, however, that program doesn't cover undocumented women like Gloria.

Worldwide, cervical cancer is the third most common cancer in women. But in the United States, it is the fourteenth most common. Cervical cancer is both preventable—with pap smears, condoms, education, and the HPV vaccine—and treatable. And the United States has done a fairly good job of funding prevention and treatment. As recently as the 1940s, cervical cancer was a top killer of women of reproductive age; the reduction in cervical cancer deaths is a major victory.

However, certain groups within the United States are still quite vulnerable to dying of cervical cancer. Latina women are diagnosed with cervical cancer at twice the rate of white women. Foreign-born Latinas are even more vulnerable. The Texas border is a cervical cancer hot spot with the highest rates in the nation. There are also racial disparities there: In some counties on the Texas border, Latina women are twice as likely to die of cervical cancer than white women living in the same county. Black women are not as likely as Latinas to be diagnosed with the disease, but black women who are diagnosed with cervical cancer are more likely to die of it than white or Latina patients.* Disparities like this—in a preventable, treatable disease—often reflect disparities in access to care. Even though screening and treatment can be funded, women without regular primary care are unlikely to be screened.

So in a sense, it was unsurprising that we found cervical cancer in Gloria. As a foreign-born, uninsured Latina woman living in poverty in Texas, she was among the people most likely to be diagnosed with this disease. Yet even though undocumented women like Gloria are the most likely to get cervical cancer, they are deliberately excluded from the programs that fund treatment.

So, we started caring for Gloria's cancer at St. Vincent's. This meant moving piecemeal through the steps of diagnosis and staging while we tried to find charity care for Gloria. Jacqueline made sure to be present at each of Gloria's appointments—the cervical biopsy, then the endometrial biopsy. If Jacqueline wasn't the student in charge, she would translate. Gloria took to hugging her, holding one of Jacqueline's hands in her own, and saying *que Dios te bendiga*—may God bless you. Meanwhile, Gloria was rejected by three hospitals in the Houston area, starting with UTMB. Every time she was rejected, Jacqueline gave her the bad news.

Jacqueline is no longer a practicing Catholic, but sometimes after these encounters she would call her father. "It will work out, Jacqueline," he said. "This is why you should go to church."

If it doesn't work out, Jacqueline thought, *I'm going to need to pray to somebody.*

As the rejections kept rolling in, Jacqueline and Gloria began cooking up more elaborate plans to get Gloria the cancer care she needed. Somehow, Jacqueline convinced St. Vincent's House to fund three thousand dollars for a CT scan to find out if Gloria had cancer in the rest of her body. One of the doctors got on Jacqueline's case for dedicating so much to this one patient. "Do you think she's trying to play you?" he asked.

* For more background on this, see the 2013 report "Latinas and Cervical Cancer in Texas: A Public Health Crisis," by the National Latina Institute for Reproductive Health.

For what? Jacqueline thought.

When the scan came back negative, showing that the cancer hadn't spread, the same doctor asked Jacqueline why, then, they had needed it. Jacqueline was just silently grateful to see that the cancer had not invaded Gloria's organs.

This took time, and in some ways it felt like we were stalling—killing time while we scratched around for someone to offer surgery and chemo. If Gloria could have been admitted to a hospital, all of these things—the biopsy, the scan, beginning treatment—could have been done in a day or two. But at St. Vincent's, weeks turned into a month, then two months. The cancer was growing. Over the course of a workday, blood seeped through Gloria's underwear.

JACQUELINE DOES NOT PARTICULARLY believe in being well-rounded as a doctor. She resents the pressure to treat medicine as a job, to leave it in the hospital. Her father never left his work at the office; he was always on call, always thinking about his patients.

"Part of me doesn't want medicine to be the way I derive meaning from life," Jacqueline said, "but that's just the way it's going to be. Why is it so bad that I want my life to have meaning from my work?"

Some part of me wanted to stop Jacqueline then, to tell her that life is full of meaning and we do not have to take it all from medicine. For a moment I saw her rushing toward a cliff that only I could see, but I couldn't stop her any more than I could stop myself. She chose medicine.

So she drove Gloria into Houston, where Gloria's application for charity care was rejected by the MD Anderson Cancer Center.

Gloria told Jacqueline to trust in God.

"Faith is amorphous," Jacqueline told me.

The worst day came when Jacqueline and Gloria were trying to figure out if Gloria could move to Houston—or fake an address in Houston—to get indigent care coverage under the Houston hospital district. But Gloria had nothing: no bills, no pay stubs, nothing that showed her address at all.

"Maybe we can get you enrolled in a study," the doctor at St. Vincent's said, lightly patting Gloria's back. Jacqueline translated, and Gloria burst into tears.

"Are you telling me I won't get care?" she said. "I'm not sure I want to go on. I want to go back to El Salvador and be with my family. I want to go back to El Salvador to die."

Jacqueline went home and keeled to the floor with guilt.

But like a miracle, the answer came the very next day. Gloria called Jacqueline on her cell phone. Thanks in large part to Jacqueline's advocacy, Gloria had been accepted to Houston Methodist for charity care. She would begin treatment the next week. She wept on the phone, and Jacqueline wept again. Gloria would not go back to El Salvador; she would stay, and live.

Sometimes medical students and doctors do get too involved with our patients; sometimes we sacrifice our family lives, our art, the things that keep us human. But sometimes when you push and push and push, and you don't give up—when you become that obsessive doctor who can think of nothing else—you actually save your patient's life.

Jacqueline and Gloria still talk on the phone sometimes, even now that Gloria has her own doctors and no longer needs to come to St. Vincent's. Gloria prays for Jacqueline, and Jacqueline meditates. Meditation doesn't feel quite full enough, though, and so sometimes she prays in a vague, earnest way. She is not quite sure whom she is praying to, but sometimes, she just needs to pray.

CHAPTER 25

ONE FEBRUARY NIGHT, LATE AFTER CLINIC, MY FELLOW
student director Julian and I were sitting on his back porch smoking
a cigar. Sarah and Dave were asleep on couches in Julian's apartment.
We four directors had all gone dancing that night, and hung out at
Julian's until Sarah and Dave conked out. The three of them were
nearly done with medical school: they would match into residency
programs the next month, and all of us would wrap up our year of
directing. In the last few months, with the incredible stress of learning to be directors and running the clinic finally easing, we had all
become close friends.

Julian passed me the cigar, then leaned back against the porch
railing and laughed again at the fact that I was smoking. He was a
military medical student, set to become a military surgeon, and the
occasional fat cigar seemed to suit him well.

"Nice," he said.

"Yeah," I said, leaning back.

"So we're almost done," he said.

"Yeah," I said. "Well, I still have to finish grad school. Are you
worried about residency?"

"Nah," he said. "I hope I get Seattle, but if I go to Walter Reed
it'll be okay."

Then we talked about being a military doctor for a while, and Julian said that he was looking forward to being deployed. He said that other people didn't understand that, why he would look forward to it, why he wouldn't just be afraid to get hurt or want to stay home in his regular life. People thought it was crazy, he said.

"Naw, it makes sense to me," I said, a bit drunkenly. "Let me tell you a story about Cicero."

Julian smiled. He was a classic military dude: brusque, a bit concrete, the kind of guy who thinks hierarchies are just great and will soon be at the top of many. But he enjoyed how Sarah and I always talked about the medical humanities; it blew his mind a little bit. He leaned back and took the cigar from me, settling in to hear my story.

"Cicero was a Roman," I began, "who lived around the year 100 BC." At the time he was alive, the Roman Empire had been in a state of constant civil war for over three hundred years. So a virtuous Roman man was always ready to serve the empire—as either statesman or soldier—and all of virtue was wrapped up in that social duty. The inner life, the emotional life, was not seen as important. In fact, it was a kind of liability. Romans were expected to present a smooth exterior face to society, and not only to outwardly appear emotionally restrained, but to actually not feel perturbed by emotion.*

But Cicero had a crisis when his beloved daughter died. He began to show his grief in public, and he had to retreat to his country estate. There, along with his friends, he wrote the Tusculan Disputations, including "On Grief of Mind," in which he argues that a virtuous man would suppress the lower, emotional, feminine side with the higher, rational, male side. And medicine has been struggling with this kind of virtue ever since. Like Cicero, we are meant to give up our lives to the service of others. But now, to serve contemporary Americans who see emotional sincerity as a virtue, we are called on to be emotionally engaged. Cicero's story reminds me that our emotional restraint (which can be mistaken for coldness) has a history and

* Robert E. Proctor, *Defining the Humanities: How Rediscovering a Tradition Can Improve Our Schools* (Bloomington: Indiana University Press, 1988).

serves a purpose: it is part of the traditional armamentarium of she who would dedicate her life to the service of others.

"So, like, I get that," I concluded. "I get why you would want to be deployed, and you're not freaking out about it or trying to stay home. Your life is actually not about your own experience. It's about serving this other thing."

Julian leaned over and put his arm around my shoulder. "Thanks, Rach," he said. "Most people don't get that."

AT TIMES, ST. VINCENT'S CLINIC seemed to shamble on without us—we directors would be at loose ends, running from room to room, or sniping at one another, but somehow miraculously all the patients were seen, the volunteers survived, and the faculty kept showing up. I came to respect the chaos of the clinic as a productive kind of chaos. You cannot try to control the thing completely. You have to trust that the clinic, which is older than I am and will endure until the need for it is over, works.

There were, as Mr. Jackson would say, many patients whom we could not get all the way to five. Jacob met a man at the Luke Society clinic one morning who had a bent forearm in a filthy splint. He'd broken his arm and gone to UTMB. The break was not complicated, so they put him in a splint and sent him home. Which would have been fine, Jacob says, if somebody had explained to him that he should not remove the splint. But he took it off to shower, and the broken ends of the bones in his arm slipped out of contact, leaving his forearm crooked and his fingers numb from a pinched nerve. Jacob began "making friends in the orthopedic surgery community," as he calls his efforts to get this patient care. The surgeons would agree to look at an X-ray, but not to correct the displaced fracture with the surgery he needed. They couldn't use an operating room without UTMB approval, as Susan well knew. So the man, who used to be a handyman, is now slightly deformed and slightly disabled, and he is a St. Vincent's patient now. Meanwhile, Jacob is still Jacob, unflappable and good, though I know he feels guilty sometimes, too. He still listens to Nine Inch Nails.

So often, our goal was to get people out of St. Vincent's and into something better. Sometimes that happened, and when it did it was often thanks to the Affordable Care Act. Mrs. Theroux, for example, had heart failure and chronic diarrhea and malignant hypertension and chronic pain, and had had two strokes so she was maintained on blood thinners that we had to check the levels on every week. She also cared for her elderly blind husband, who always seemed so joyful when he answered the phone and I said it was me calling from St. Vincent's. "Thank you so much for all y'all do," he would say, so that I could feel his smile warming me through the telephone line. Well, Mrs. Theroux finally got insurance. "Thank the good Lord," she said, and I was grateful, too. She died not long after, but she did not lack love and care in this world.

But the Affordable Care Act never helped us in the way it was supposed to. It never made St. Vincent's obsolete: first, because it deliberately excluded undocumented people from getting coverage, and second, because Texas did not expand Medicaid. Our patients were mostly the working poor—white, brown, black, whomever—and most of them would qualify for Medicaid if Texas would expand it. At the time of this writing, 17 percent of Texans are still uninsured, including 11 percent of children.* Medicaid expansion would help a lot. It is the low-hanging fruit of health policy, supported by the Texas Medical Association and basically everyone else with common sense. But it still wouldn't make St. Vincent's obsolete.

And it was always so pleasant to practice there, even with the pain and the frustration. It was good to do medicine in a place that felt perfectly embedded in the community, as if the clinic were a natural outgrowth of the neighborhood. It was good to know that my patients were all welcome there; indeed, they were *expected*. It was

---

* For reasonably up-to-date statistics on insurance coverage in Texas and other states, see the U.S. Census Bureau at www.census.gov or the Kaiser Family Foundation at www.kff.org.

good to hear all the sounds of life—basketballs thumping, kids on the playground, guys on the street happily shouting back and forth—in that moment at the beginning of a physical exam when I would close my eyes to feel my patient's heartbeat pulsing up through his or her wrist.

St. Vincent's gave me so much. The knowledge that the clinic should not exist, that every one of my patients deserved something more, hung always in the background, even as the clinic became the largest piece of my heart.

Once upon a time, I was preoccupied with who I might become in medical school. I thought I was an artist, and I thought I needed to fight against the forces that would try to socialize me into medicine—to deaden me, to numb me, to make me cool and objective. So fight I did, with a haughtiness that nearly cost me some friendships. But ultimately, medicine won.

Medicine changed me, but not in the ways I expected. It became for me what Susan sought when she joined the profession: a total identity. I know that's probably difficult to understand. But I think often of Jacqueline's question—"Why is it so bad that I want my life to have meaning from my work?"—and my answer is that it isn't bad at all. It's exactly who a doctor should be.

I have a life, of course. I have a dog, I go camping, I plant a pathetic garden every spring that dies in August. I could no more separate my medical identity from my identity as a person or as a writer than I could separate the earth from the sky. And—even with the paperwork and the injustice and the hassle—I could imagine no life more meaningful than the life I have been able to live through medicine and through St. Vincent's. It is the life I wanted, in the end: It is solid. It is real. The trick is to give up, and let medicine become you.

SEVEN YEARS AFTER THE HURRICANE, Susan tells me that very little has changed. "This is not a happy story," she says. "This is still not a happy, good story."

Her house-call bag, the one she carried out to Beaumont so many times, is still on a shelf in her garage. She is still having the same conversations with unfunded patients; she is still doggedly applying to Casebook. Her patients are routinely rejected but she feels that it's important to try, so that somehow the need, and the need's refusal, can be documented. More good people have left UTMB, and some in heartbreak, but many remain. Susan tells the St. Vincent's directors that, if we ever need a faculty member to cover, she lives ten minutes from the clinic and she'll just drive over.

After her Ike experience, Susan became board certified in hospice and palliative medicine. Having cared for so many dying patients in their homes, she was eligible for the "practice pathway"—that is, she achieved board certification without having to do a fellowship. She never expected to become a palliative care physician, but the work compels her, and now she both practices surgery and cares for the dying.

"I almost can't remember what I thought doctoring would be like," she says, "because it has been so different. And it was so characterized by that sudden loss of ability to doctor, when all those patients were lost."

In April, I passed off my keys to Jacqueline. My year of directing had wound to its end, and it was time for me to go take care of other things. "These were Htin's keys," I said. "This is the key to the banana room. This is the key to the chapel. This is the key to the medication closet in the hallway. This is the key to the counseling room." I went on and on.

"There's no way I'm going to remember all these," Jacqueline said.

"I know," I told her. "It's totally overwhelming. But you'll be fine."

EPILOGUE

SOMETIMES I DREAM OF MEETING MR. ROSE AGAIN. THIS is not a dream I have at night, but a daydream. In it, we are back at St. Vincent's in the sweltering Galveston summer, and he is himself then but I am who I have become now. In the dream, I get it right. I think clearly and systematically like a physician, instead of being baffled by his illness. I dig deeper, slow down, ask more questions. If in the dream I make a mistake, I am able to explain it and apologize. And if in the dream he is still dying, I stand by his side. I visit him in the hospital; I get to know his family.

In the daydream, sometimes I am so good that I am able to take his pain away, or to finagle a late-breaking, miraculous cure for him. Other times it is more realistic: I cannot make the cup of suffering pass from him. But I am able to sit with him a while longer in that hospital room, to breathe in deeply of his suffering and offer what I can of my compassion. I am able to apologize.

At times I even feel compassion for my poor baffled medical student self. I was early in my training, and I was trying so hard to help. I made a mistake, and I needed—for my own human reasons—to apologize. I lost my chance to do so because I didn't have the guts, or the grace, to return to visit my patient. I know now that returning to be with those who are suffering is no easy thing. I also know that it is my job.

I can only apologize to the sky now. I am sorry.

ACKNOWLEDGMENTS

I am grateful to, and humbled by, the patients who have so gracefully allowed me to be part of their care. Thanks to Mr. Michael Jackson and the whole community at St. Vincent's, particularly my crop of directors: Sarah Baker, Toug Tanavin, Julian Vellucci, Roxi Radi, Kelli Gross, Sean Kelly, Lauren Fuez, Samantha Dorer, Jamie Hinderliter, and Suzanne Snow. One of our group, David Gersztenkorn, passed away before this book was published; his death was a loss to us all.

My research mentor Jason E. Glenn opened my eyes to many of the structural and social issues that emerge in this book. I am grateful to him and to all those at the Institute for the Medical Humanities who helped form me as a scholar and humanist.

Many thanks to my first and best mentor in writing, Michael Adams. Also to Forrest Wilder and all the folks at the *Texas Observer*, for keeping the Great State on its toes. Thanks to my excellent agent, Zoë Pagnamenta, for seeing this work through from scratch. I am grateful for the sharp editorial guidance of John Glusman at Norton, and all the folks there who have contributed so much to this book.

I'm grateful to all those who have taught me medicine, but particularly to Susan McCammon, Robert Beach, Patricia Beach, Howard Brody, Michael Boyars, Bruce Russell, Adrian Billings, and Serena Aunon. Thanks as always to the John P. McGovern Academy for Oslerian Medicine, for crucial financial and moral support during my medical education.

And of course my friends, especially Delaney Hall, Caitlin Sweetlamb, Graham Schmidt, Katherine Strandberg, Freddie Joseph, Christina Gomez-Mira, Ryan Kiesler, Amerisa Waters, Katie Ray, Margaret Wardlaw, and Parth Gejji. Thanks to the Historic Pleasure Palace, the Big Yellow House in the Sky, and all the physicians and scientists who shared their homes and years with me.

And of course my family. And Ben Laussade, my lantern on the trail.

INDEX

Note: Many of the names in the index are pseudonyms.